'Beautifully written with u
and Far Away is an intricate
the power of memory. I cou
            Lisa

'What a beautiful book! I love   ...ies journey as a young man with the wonderful Alf by his side, and as an old man with his family around him as his memories begin to fracture. His granddaughter, Nina, is a breath of fresh air and the scenes with both her and Ernie are the most warming and humorous. *The Everyday and Far Away* is a poignant and heartbreaking tale, but it has an ending that will leave you feeling incredibly uplifted and joyous.'

Kate Galley, author of *Old Girls Behaving Badly*

'This charming novel about characters with dementia and ADHD is more than the sum of its parts. I was moved to tears by its quiet beauty and layered characters.'

Laura Pearson, author of *The Last List of Mabel Beaumont*

'One of those rare novels that will burrow right inside your heart and nestle there forever... I cried more tears over the tragedy and love rendered in this story than I think I ever have in a novel. Dementia is a difficult subject, but Jones handles it with perfection, never sentimental or patronising, but with a raw, emotional truth.'

Louise Fein, author of *People Like Us*

'A thoroughly heartwarming and deeply moving story. It's so beautifully written, with characters I grew to adore, and the soul-stirring ending left me smiling through tears.'

Lisa Timoney, author of *His Secret Wife*

'This is a story about the extraordinary lives of ordinary people. I haven't read a book that's touched me so deeply in a long, long time. Jones takes you on an incredibly emotional journey with a deftness of touch.'

Victoria Scott, author of *The Women Who Wouldn't Leave*

JACQUELINE JONES lives in Guildford and *The Everyday and Far Away* is her first novel in this genre. As Jacqueline Sutherland she writes psychological suspense, and she is currently at work on a romance series under the name Pippa Nixon.

The Everyday and Far Away

JACQUELINE JONES

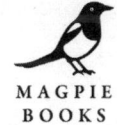

MAGPIE
BOOKS

A MAGPIE BOOK

First published in Great Britain, the Republic of Ireland and Australia
by Magpie, an imprint of Oneworld Publications Ltd, 2025

Copyright © Jacqueline Jones, 2025

The moral right of Jacqueline Jones to be identified as the
Author of this work has been asserted by her in accordance
with the Copyright, Designs and Patents Act 1988

All rights reserved
Copyright under Berne Convention
A CIP record for this title is available from the British Library

ISBN 978-0-86154-964-1
eISBN 978-0-86154-963-4

Printed and bound in Great Britain by Clays Ltd, Elcograf S.p.A.

This book is a work of fiction. Names, characters, businesses,
organisations, places and events are either the product of the author's
imagination or are used fictitiously. Any resemblance to actual
persons, living or dead, events or locales is entirely coincidental.

No part of this publication may be reproduced, stored in a retrieval system, or
transmitted, in any form or by any means, electronic, mechanical, photocopying,
recording or otherwise, without the prior permission of the publishers.

The authorised representative in the EEA is eucomply OÜ,
Pärnu mnt 139b–14, 11317 Tallinn, Estonia
(email: hello@eucompliancepartner.com / phone: +33757690241)

Oneworld Publications Ltd
10 Bloomsbury Street
London WC1B 3SR
England

Stay up to date with the latest books,
special offers, and exclusive content from
Oneworld with our newsletter

Sign up on our website
oneworld-publications.com

For my mum, in the everyday,
and my dad, in the far away,
with all my love.

Prologue

1969

Stephen's aim was way off. The first two balls weren't even in the vicinity of the coconut; one went wide and one fell short. His face was the picture of concentration as he sized up the target again, but I wondered whether the coconut would fall off even if he did manage to hit it straight and true. He rubbed the third and final ball in his little hands before closing one eye and poking his tongue out the corner of his mouth. He didn't do any kind of convoluted run-up as we'd seen some others do while he waited his turn, he just pulled his five-year-old arm back as far as he could and threw the ball with a grunt at the coconut shy. The ball – miraculously – chipped the coconut and it wobbled, everyone "oohed", but it stayed sitting on its stick, as though glued in position, which it probably was. All the spectators "aaahed" and the next child stepped up to lose his money.

Phyllis swept in with a hug and a "never mind", leaving me to mind the pushchair. Susie sat inside like the Queen, pointing chubby fingers at the things she wanted to see. Her cheeks were rosy in the chill of a spring that hadn't found its heat yet. She grinned at me, and waved vaguely towards the flashing lights of the helter-skelter. I winked at her and she drooled in return.

Phyllis and I had been coming to the fair together for seven years. The first time we came, we took the Ferris wheel and she clutched my arm every time we rode over the top, laughing out loud. By the time we'd done three rounds, my arm was round her shoulder and you couldn't fit a cigarette paper between us. The following year, we'd ridden it as man and wife. The town spread out below us like a million different opportunities.

Now, Phyllis manoeuvred the pushchair over the grass towards the swing-boats and carousels.

Stephen trotted in front, unperturbed at not having a coconut. He didn't like them anyway – he'd tried them when we first got them in at the shop. He half-ran, half-skipped, checking back over his shoulder every now and then to make sure we were following.

Alf and Peggy the Pie came out of the bustle towards us, both carrying a bag with a goldfish inside. They bent to Susie for her to see. She squealed and reached out the wet hand she'd been sucking on.

"You haven't, Alf." Phyllis laughed, "Not again!"

Alf straightened himself up, gently moving the bag away from Susie's fingers that were trying to squeeze the fish through the plastic.

"Keston Ponds could always do with a few more," he said, which was where most of the fair fish ended up. Some of them were almost a foot long now. "Want to help me tomorrow, Stephen? We can set them free?" He mussed the boy's hair and Stephen nodded, but his eyes were already straining ahead towards the rides.

"We're heading back," said Peggy the Pie, tightening her headscarf under her chin against the wind.

"Might stop off at The Sovereigns on the way?" Alf suggested to test her reaction and, at her agreeable nod, they were soon swallowed again by the crowd, waving over their shoulders as they went. We pushed on, through the smells of hot dogs and strains of tinny music, until we reached the carousel, where Stephen had stopped and hopped foot to foot, his mouth open in wonder.

I rubbed the coins together in my trouser pocket, thinking about the candyfloss we'd shared and games we'd tried. The ride on the dodgems for Stephen and me, jolting and laughing our way around the rink. Throwing darts onto playing cards trying to pin a king. Tossing ping-pong balls into a bucket in the hope of winning a toy car. Finally, the coconut shy. My coins felt few and small between my fingers. Stephen turned to me and his eyes shone in hope.

Susie wailed, fed up of sitting so long, and Phyllis lumped her out of the pushchair and up onto her hip, much to Susie's delight. She immediately stuck her sticky fingers into Phyl's ear.

I shuffled the pennies in my hand and looked at the sign hanging on the fence advertising the price.

Stephen appeared in front of me, bouncing up and down.

"Please can I have a go, Dad? Please."

"Have we got enough?" Phyl whispered, disengaging her earlobe from Sue. I surveyed the money in my palm. It would mean no pint at The Sovereigns on the way home.

"We have," I said decisively, taking the two steps forward and pressing the coins into the fair man's outstretched hand.

Stephen pulled on my arm, with a "thank-you" and then whooped and ran, not chancing a change of mind. He scooted up the metal steps and round the platform to the other side of the carousel, out of sight.

"Do you think he needs help?" Phyllis said, wrinkling her brow, "do you think it's safe?"

"He'll be fine. He's a big boy," I said, craning my neck to spot him, but the central column blocked our view and all we could do was wait.

The music started and the carousel lurched into life. Creaking metal, flashing lights. The excited shriek of children as the ride began. A candy-pink horse went by with a small girl clutching its plastic mane. An older boy passed next in an aeroplane too small for him, his knees tucked up under his chin. I recognised next the children from down the road, riding a fire engine together. One rang the rope bell so continuously that the other one turned round and punched him on the arm. Then, a teacup on a saucer, a grey elephant and a police car. Eventually Stephen came into view. He'd chosen a red motorbike and his grin split his face in two as he leaned into the corner. He pretended to rev the grips and he waved as he rode past.

"Ha!" Phyllis chuckled, bouncing Susie on her hip. "Should have known. Just like his dad."

And I could sense the smile on my face was just as big as Stephen's and realised it was the best few pennies I'd ever spent.

The Everyday

"You used to love going out on your motorbike, didn't you Dad?"

My beer was almost gone. I swilled my jar and flicked a hopeful look towards the waiter. If he came over, Phyllis might take the hint and get me another one. It was Sunday after all. I swallowed the last mouthful and smacked my lips.

"Eh, Dad?"

The two women were looking at me. Phyllis, best blue cardigan on, and Sue, blotchy red from the heat of the fire. Nina was the only one not staring at me; her eyes were glued to the phone in her hand that beeped and chirruped quietly.

"I said, you used to love riding your bike?"

Eyebrows up, voice raised. Don't know when she started talking to me as though I was deaf. Like I'm some old codger. Bloody cheek. Mind you, she's knocking on herself a bit now. Who would have thought I'd have a middle-aged daughter with kids – and grandkids – of her own? Not my little Susie any more. More like Solid Sue by the look of the extra pounds she'd managed to squeeze into her jeans recently. Not that I'm allowed to comment on anything like that. More than my life is worth. In fact, there's lots of things I'm not supposed to say apparently. "They're out of date," she says.

"We just don't say things like that, Dad," she'd said before. "Specially not in public."

Public? We were only at the Rose and Crown. And I'd been drinking in there since before she was a gleam in my eye. Wasn't like I was on stage or something, was it? Silly bugger.

But they're still looking at me. Waiting. Oh, yes. The motorbike.

"A Norton, wasn't it?" Sue said.

I wiped my mouth on the back of my hand and Phyllis passed me a napkin.

"Norton Dominator," I said and it came out a bit gruff, on the back of the roast beef and a jug of gravy. "A beauty." I rubbed my hands together, sat back in my chair.

Sue rubbed the last piece of Yorkshire pudding around the plate, soaking up any last drop of meat juice. Good appetite she had, my girl. Her fork glinted silver in the light as she chewed and it reminded me of the chrome of my twin cylinders, the shine of my handlebars.

"Made in 1953. Saved all my wages in the service for almost two years before I picked her up. It's important to save for things."

"I know, Dad," she said through the batter. "Like you always told us. A third to the rent. A third to live on. And—"

"Third to savings." I sniffed and nodded. Seems like she did listen to me after all.

"Took a trip to the coast at the weekend," I said. "Ran like a dream."

Sue threw a quick glance at Phyllis, who shrugged just an inch without raising her eyes, painstakingly cutting the last piece of chicken into two equal pieces, small enough to nibble. She was a dainty eater, my Phyl, ladylike.

The motorbike really had gone like a charm. Engine never missed a tick. Wheels held the tarmac like glue. I'd not taken the motorway, that's no way to travel. Enjoyed the scenic route all the way. A roads and back lanes. Where the traffic was lighter, and the verges made a green soft shoulder along your side. It was one of those spring days that had no heat in it, but enough brightness to tempt the bulbs out the ground. Mile after mile of fields around me, the wind on my cheeks under my goggles. Helmet strap flapping under my chin. Bike engine thrumming between my thighs. Road under my wheels. The feeling inside that couldn't be beat. In fact, the only thing that would make it better would be the thing I'd never done. Ride without a helmet. Blessed as I was with ears that grew outwards like two handles off my head, the press of the helmet held them trapped and sore. Maybe one day, I'd do it. To feel the wind on my face and ears. Just the once. When no one was looking. But probably not, I know more than most how quickly accidents can happen.

"When I filled her up, a fella came over to stare," I said to Susie. He had too, a man in his fifties maybe, leaned on the pump while I screwed the petrol cap back on. Nodded his appreciation when I turned the key and the engine kicked straight in. He obviously knew quality when he saw it.

"But I thought—" Sue said, and Phyllis shook her head, just once, and then speared the last bit of chicken.

I picked up my pint for a sup but it was empty. I must have finished it. Glanced about for the waiter and luck was with me. The nearest boy looked my way and I waved my jar at him, getting a salute in return. Nina saw what I was doing and I threw her a wink. She bit her lip to keep herself quiet and grinned back. She was a good one, was Nina. My favourite. Another thing I wasn't allowed to say. She had the busiest brain I ever knew and sometimes she had trouble keeping up with it. But she'd get there.

"Little Freddie's apparently got a football match at school this weekend, Mum, if you want to come?" Sue was off onto the next thing. She was always changing subject, one to the other, sometimes left me behind and then tutted that I wasn't keeping up. Didn't give me time to draw breath. "Nina can mind the shop for a few hours, can't you, Neen? Mind you, after what happened last time I left her on her own—"

"Mum, do you have to?" Nina cut in, rolling her eyes in her mum's direction.

"Left a delivery of cabbages out in the yard and the pigeons ruined the lot."

"MUM!" Nina hissed as Sue tried a little laugh, even though it didn't sound like she found it very funny. "Anyway," Sue carried on, turning to Phyllis again. "Can you come?"

"That'd be nice, love. Long as Dad's having a good day." Phyllis put her knife and fork together quietly.

Sue was chatting about directions, and football boots and the like, but it was of no interest to me. I was still remembering the smell of the sea through my visor that told me I was only a few miles away from the Witterings. The vibration of the road under my wheels. The lean of the bike on the corner. All the things that you never got in a car. The things that, unless you've been on a bike, you'd never understand.

From the first time I rode pillion with Alf, I wanted a motorbike of my own. And after I went solo on Alf's bike, I never looked back. Must have only been about eighteen, just before I went in the army for my national service. And then I got one there to ride too. A BSA M20, it was. 500cc. Heavy-framed with a low-end torque, it must have been good in the war for getting up and down the hills and bumps of the battlefield. Not that I saw any of that, mind. My hands were fair shaking when I got off after that first time, but my blood pulsed around like I could hear it. After that, I was sold.

"Here you go, Ernie," the waiter said and put a fresh jar in front of me.

"Thanks, lad," I said, taking quick hold on the handle.

"When did he order that?" Sue said to Phyllis, who blew the air out of her lips in a half raspberry, chuckling.

I grinned and took a long pull. Under the frothy head, it was good and cold and I felt it all the way down.

"Might as well have another one myself then," said Sue, but, when the waiter looked expectantly at Phyllis, she shook her head and eyed her small glass of wine, almost untouched still on the table.

"Looks like you're in for a quiet afternoon, Mum," Sue said when the waiter brought her wine back, a large, I noticed. She got that from me. I liked a tipple. When I was allowed, that was. Phyllis was always watching me like a hawk these days. Moaning about how it got in the way of my pills. Took so many of them in the mornings now, I must rattle. But maybe she was letting me have a day off, because she smiled in my direction and said, "Two pints will have you snoring in your armchair, love." I tipped my glass at her. My girls, a pint and a nap. Sounded good to me.

Sue and Phyllis started talking quietly between themselves. Every now and then one of them glanced at me, as if checking I was still there. Silly buggers. Where else was I going to be? Nina was kicking her feet under the table, bored. I supped my pint and turned my chair towards the fire.

Nothing better than an open fire. We'd had one in number 31 where I grew up. Dot and I used to sit in front of it and spit on the wood to hear it hiss. She always ended up with dribble on her chin. She wasn't a very good spitter, Our Dot. Maybe because she only had baby teeth. Dinky Dot I used to call her. Mam used to smack the tops of our heads as she walked past if she caught us playing that game.

"What did the doctor say when you rang then?" Sue said and I smiled at her, thinking about Dot and her gappy grin, and then went back to the fire. It was dying down a bit. I heaved myself out of my chair to the hearth and used the poker hanging there to stoke it. Fresh sparks flew from under the logs, like little fireworks. Whizz bangs, Dot called them. I gave it another prod, got a good bit of air under the wood, until a new flame licked upwards.

"Wants to do some tests," Phyllis said. Was she ill? I fixed her with a look, but she seemed all right. Bit flushed maybe, but that would be the wine. She always got a little red when she drank. It started at her collar and crept up. She saw me looking and smiled. She was fine.

Hanging the poker back on its nail, I let myself drop back in the chair to finish my pint. The fire had picked up nicely and I stretched my legs towards it. Not a bad way to spend a Sunday. Unless it was the first Sunday of the month. Then I had other places to be.

"Just so forgetful…" Phyllis said.

"Who's forgetful?" I asked but they both ignored me. Maybe they couldn't remember. Ha. I smiled at my own wit and was going to tell them but they were deep in conversation. Girl talk, obviously. I decided it was time for a quick visit to the loo. The second pint suddenly making its presence felt. I hoisted myself up and out of the chair and set off to the toilets. At least they were inside these days. No running off out the back of the house.

By the time I got back, I knew there was no chance of another pint as Phyllis was already buttoning up her coat. Sue said she was paying the bill this week, but I said, "over my dead body," and handed my wallet to Phyllis to count out the money. There's certain things that are just not right. And your own children paying the bill is one of them.

"Thanks, Dad," she said, then, "Let's get you home." I let her pull my jacket on and then she gave me a little squeeze as she zipped it up. She smelled nice and it was a soft kind of hug, what with her having quite a lot of fat on her. Nina bounced foot to foot beside her, desperate to get out. I felt the same all of a sudden.

"Back to my bike," I said, rubbing my hands together. I might give her a bit of a polish this afternoon; buff her till I could see my face in the chrome.

I went first, leading the way for my girls. My wife, my daughter, my youngest granddaughter. I was a lucky man. The waiter opened the door for me and saluted as I went through.

"See you next week, Ernie," he said as the cold air hit me.

"If you're lucky," I said back and he laughed.

Sue and Phyllis pulled their coats round them tight as they came out behind me. Nina pulled her hood up so that all I could see was her nose to her chin. Phyllis clutched her car keys like she was scared she was going to lose them.

"Over there," she said and pointed at our car as though I didn't know which one it was.

"I know, woman," I said and set off in the direction of the car park.

"Still going on about his motorbike then?" Sue asked behind me.

"Sitting in the garage collecting dust," Phyllis said. "Hasn't ridden it in years."

I aimed for a small red car and trudged towards it until a hand on my elbow steered me towards a different one.

"I know, I know," I said, but I didn't really.

Nina

Sunday lunch torture.

"Keep your feet still, Nina, you're jiggling the table." Mum nodded at the cutlery vibrating in time to her toe tapping.

Nina moved her thigh so that it no longer rested against the table leg but continued to jiggle, silently, invisibly under her chair where it wouldn't bother anyone. Mum went back to Nan's story and Nina picked at the skin round her fingernail. The sore bit.

They'd been there hours, surely. She snuck a glance at the clock on the heavily patterned wallpaper of the pub and was surprised to see it was only 1.30p.m. so they hadn't actually been there that long at all. And it wasn't as if she had something better to do anyway. She exhaled, as quietly as she could. Not that Nan and Pops would notice, but Mum had ears like a bat and could hear a sigh at five metres. If they'd let her have her phone again she could play a game and distract herself but Mum had put it in her bag and buckled it shut.

It wasn't that Nina didn't like Sunday lunch with Nan and Pops, as she did. Especially her pops, whose eyes twinkled when he talked of motorbikes. It was just they ate so slowly. The pace of their eating made her antsy. Maybe it was the lack of true teeth. Perhaps falsies had a speed restriction on them, like some of the delivery lorries she saw on the way to college. The thought of college made her jiggle faster and Sue threw her a look over her roast beef, one eyebrow raised. Nina bit her lip and slowed her foot again. Her mum went back to talking to Nan, telling her the latest in the shop. The shortage of strawberries due to the earlier cold weather. While they were talking she saw her pops motion to the waiter for another pint. She grinned at him and he winked at her to keep quiet. She nodded and sipped her fizzy water, Mum's latest solution to her problems.

"Let's try cutting out the sugar, Neen," Sue had said, as tactfully as she could the month before. Nina always knew her mum's different voices. This one was the "I might sound like I'm making a suggestion but I strongly advise you do it" tone. "It can be linked to hyperactivity, you know."

So now she was not only hyperactive but so full of water that she had to pee every hour. At least it gave her an excuse to get up from her chair. The thought of getting up now made her jiggle faster and she reached into her hoodie pocket for her fidget spinner. A palm-sized pink metal flower that her mum had bought her, in bulk, from the internet.

"That way, you can keep one in your pocket, or in the car, or in your bedroom, or in your…"

Nina had nodded. She got the point. She was not just annoying to her mum in one place, she was annoying people everywhere. She couldn't help it. It was the way she was made. When she was younger, people used to call her a "live wire" or an "energetic child". Now she was obviously just irritating.

"How's college going, Nina?" her nan asked, finally putting her knife and fork together on her clean plate.

Nina began to spin the gadget in her fingers, flick, flick, flick as she considered how to answer.

"It's off to a good start isn't it, love?" Sue said with an overly bright smile, which was not what she'd said the night before when Nina's tutor rang to discuss her progress. "Although her teacher did tell me she needs to pay more attention."

"You daydreaming again, Nina?" said her nan, not unkindly. It had been a running joke for years about school reports, but one which everyone was finding less and less funny. Most of all, Nina. Her older sister Jess always got the As and Bs. Though school was long gone for her and now she was focused on getting a place for her own daughter, Daisy, at the same school as Freddie next year. Nina's big brother Josh always got the sports cup at the end of the year when he was at school and now he had gone on to be a personal trainer at the local gym. Nina got the "Must Try Harder"s. Or "Too Easily Distracted". Every time.

Nina breathed out, shook her head and then nodded.

"Just finding it a bit hard to concentrate on one thing at a time, Nan," she admitted.

"Cos you've got so much going on in there," her pops said proudly, tapping the side of his head above his sticky-out ears. "More brains than I ever had."

Nina wished that were true. She worried her brains didn't work at all. They never seemed to take anything in. She'd write something down and then forget what she'd written. She'd put her hand up to answer a question and then forget what the question was in the first place. Attention Deficit Hyperactivity Disorder. That's what it was. Her brain was noisy and distracted and forgetful. The only thing her brains were good at were puzzles. That was because one nice little side effect of ADHD was hyper-focus. Her grandad bought her a Rubik's cube when she was seven and she mastered it in two days. He bought her a thousand-piece jigsaw when she was eight and she sat for four hours solid and then it was done. Now she spent the Saturday wages she earned working at the family fruit and veg shop on second-hand boxes of Lego off the internet. She made magnificent scenes and homes from the pieces, complete with interiors and light switches, and sofas and logs on the fire. Activities, like Lego, could keep her attention. Sometimes, surprisingly, for hours at a time. If only she could hyper-focus on her homework or essays in the same way she might be all right. But Mum didn't know the half of it. College was NOT going well so far. Nina spun her spinner ferociously under the table, the little pink flower a whir on her palm. It made her feel a little better inside.

It was all so frustrating. Nina knew her mum was right but it wasn't like she wasn't trying. She really was. She focused as fiercely as she could on her tutors but it just wasn't that easy to hear anything over the chatter already in her head.

Nina had chosen the subjects that she liked the most from school to study at college so it should – by rights – be better than school. Although she couldn't really say she liked these subjects the most. She just hated them less than the others. So now she studied English literature, geography and sport, which her mum thought was an excellent choice because it would give her "the chance to be a bit more active". True. One of the lessons each week was a practical where her brain actually quietened down a bit while she ran about, but the others were theory-based and she jiggled under tables trying to understand the muscular system or learn about doping laws. English literature was a lot of sitting, and essays, which were a special kind of torture, and geography was no longer just learning about volcanoes and rivers. The vocabulary was not going in and every time she got asked a question in class she drew a blank. She must try harder. She must just CONCENTRATE. But her brain wasn't keen.

"Why didn't you give me a name that started with a J?" Nina asked Sue, who was mid-conversation about strawberries and took a moment to take the question in. "Like you did with Jess and Josh?"

"What? Oh…" Sue shook her head as if to clear it and then said, "Times had changed I guess… you know, names move on. Fashions changed a lot in the ten years between your sister and brother being born and then you."

"Was I an accident then?" Nina asked, knee bouncing.

Sue laughed. "More of a surprise, I'd say."

"But wasn't there a popular name beginning with J in 2001 that you could have called me?" Nina persisted.

"I called you Nina after Nina Simone, the greatest singer of all time," Mum said, lifting her glass in a silent salute to her dead icon.

"You could have called me Janina, then," Nina said, in a sudden flash of inspiration.

"Don't you like your name, love?" asked Sue, frowning and obviously wondering where this was coming from.

"It's not that," Nina said. "I just wondered why I'm not the same as the others."

"I never really thought about it," her mum said, with a little laugh, and turned back to her strawberry conversation.

Nina wondered briefly whether she'd get better school reports if her name started with a J.

Pops was pushing himself up from the chair. He launched off in the direction of the toilets and she watched the other drinkers smile and acknowledge him as he passed. Everyone knew him in the Rose and Crown. He'd been drinking in here for years. When she walked through the crowded canteen at college nobody gave her a second look. The only people that got looked at were the sporty ones who wore fancy branded tracksuits or the pretty ones with fake eyelashes and straightened hair. She didn't really make an impression one way or the other. She tried to talk to people but sometimes she saw the very slight raise of an eyebrow or eye-roll between girls and then she'd make an excuse and move on. It was hard trying to be normal. Easier to pull her hood up and stay out of it.

Her chair screeched on the floorboards as she stood up too quickly, making her nan clasp her chest theatrically.

"Where's the fire?" Nan asked, looking about, and Nina laughed.

"Sorry, Nan," she said. "Toilet time. It's all this water." She indicated her empty glass and headed towards the ladies, resisting the urge to run.

"I don't know what goes through her head, sometimes," she heard Sue say in her "where does that girl get her ideas from" way as she left. "Janina indeed."

On the way back, Nina stopped for a moment to write her name on the chalkboard next to the dartboard, doodling elaborate swirls around the letters, shading in the capital N. Anything to keep her away from the table for another five minutes.

"That's nice," Pops said, appearing behind her, and she passed him the chalk.

ernie he wrote next to her name, the chalk a bit shaky and no capital on the E. He added a big bubble dot over the i and nodded to himself in appreciation.

They surveyed their handiwork silently and then Ernie drew an apple and Nina added a smiley face. Looked like neither of them were in a rush to rejoin the others.

"So how is college?" he asked, without looking at her. "Really?"

She sighed and didn't try to hide it.

"That good, eh?" he said, drawing what she guessed was a bunch of bananas. Or at least, she HOPED they were meant to be bananas.

"What about you, Pops? How are you?"

He held the stub of chalk in his fingers and studied it for a moment.

"Apparently I'm forgetting stuff I've learned," he said, passing the white stick back to her. She held his eye, considering.

"That's not so bad," she said. "I can't even learn stuff to forget."

He laughed and put the chalk back on the shelf.

"You'll be fine, TillyMint," he said, his old nickname for her. Said it came from his childhood and now it made her eyes hot. "Keep calm and carrot on." He nudged her with his elbow and then said, "Just got to find your way."

And that, Nina thought, was the problem. She had no idea which way was hers.

"Like I did on my motorbike," he added as they walked together back to the table.

The Far Away

1944

I remember the first motorbike that ever came to our house.

I was out with the other kids in the street, knowing I could go no further than the corner and the top or Mam would be out after me and pinch my ear. She'd only done it once before when I followed the big boys to the dock road, but it went so red she kissed it a hundred times before bed and I let her think it hurt more than it really did so that she kept kissing.

"You're only four, Ernie. You stay where I can see you. I don't need to be worrying about you and all."

After that she'd test me out occasionally, appearing on the doorstep in her pinny and looking left and right double-quick to catch me if I was out of range. I can still see her giving me a little nod and a smile when I was right there, in the street in front of the red brick terrace.

I liked being out with the other kids. We played Stuck in the Mud, or British Bulldog from one pavement to the other. We ran and flew with outstretched arms and bombed Hitler into the gutter. We built a barrier with an old bed frame that the big boys dragged from the tip that we could hide behind to throw pretend grenades. I was the best at machine gun noises and Tommy Morgan was good at air-raid sirens. So good that once old Mrs Walker from number 52 put on her coat and hat and set off for the shelter. Tommy's mam had to go after her and bring her back.

There were a few of us, I forget how many, from Divine Street and Welbeck Road, brothers and sisters and their cousins and me. I sometimes wondered how they all fit in their houses. I knew their homes were all the same size as mine. Two beds upstairs. Living room with a kitchen corner downstairs. Toilet out the back but Mam let me wee in the potty at night-time or if there was frost on the doorstep. Some of my friends had so many brothers and sisters there'd be five or six of them in a bed or a room, although some of them were sharing with their mam now their dad was away. I had a bed to myself, a whole one. And so did Mam, a bigger one, till Dad came back. And I could sit by the fire and rest my back against Mam's legs as she sat in the chair in the evening. She'd stroke my head and not have to take time off for anyone else's petting. I was happy with that. I couldn't remember any other way. I couldn't even remember having to share her with Dad.

That day in Divine Street I was teasing Billy Sankey's dog with a stick when a sound got my attention. It was a slow putt-putt-putt, like it was pottering along, looking for something, unusual enough in the street. Most people walked in and out from the docks or to the market. A few rode their pushbikes to a factory or a shop. So this engine had us all looking as soon as we heard it.

And a silver motorbike made its way into the top of Welbeck Street and pulled to the kerb. Taking his chance when I wasn't paying attention, Billy's dog jumped up and grabbed the stick in his mouth, growling enough to put you off if you didn't know him. I let him have it anyway and wiped my slobbery hands on my shorts, watching as the rider lifted his goggles and rested them on his cap; he looked like something off a postcard. Leaning on one foot, he steadied himself and the bike while he pulled an

The Everyday and Far Away

envelope out of his satchel and frowned at the front, then glanced at the nearest door to read the number. The dog nudged my hand with the stick, but I pushed him away.

I edged a bit nearer. The bike wasn't out of bounds, just there on the corner, but I checked Mam wasn't at the door just in case. The bike had a big round headlight and a shiny metal middle. I'd never been so close to one before and shuffled closer again. The saddle was at my shoulders, the handlebars at my head. I stuffed my hands in my pockets to stop myself touching it. He might tell me off.

"What number you after?" Billy Sankey said, sidling up beside me. He was always the one with the chat, did the talking for all of us when there was a grown-up about. If I was known for my ears, sticking out the sides of my head, Billy Sankey was known for his gob. The man looked at his envelope again.

"Thirty-one."

"That's you, Ernie." Billy elbowed me in the ribs and the man turned to me. He pursed his lips together as though thinking and I saw he had just the start of a moustache, dark on his lip but fluffy. He wasn't quite a grown-up after all. I couldn't believe how lucky he was to have a motorbike like that.

I stuck my hand out towards the envelope to take it to Mam but he shook his head. Instead he turned the key and the engine cut out and quietened with a tick, tick, tick. He swung his leg over the bike and kicked out a metal stand on the side to lean it on. I could see my face reflected in the shine and was now standing close enough to feel the heat off the engine. The air smelled of oil and excitement, and I had a funny feeling in my tummy.

"You keep an eye on the bike for me," the man said, looking straight at me. Some of the other boys groaned out loud and Billy

Sankey said, "I could do that, Mister." I could only blink, but I managed to nod, so he knew I'd heard. My head felt like it was going to blow off with the responsibility. Me. He chose me.

I didn't even watch him walk up the street to our door. I heard him knock in the background, one, two, three but I was listening more closely to the tiny sounds of the engine cooling, the tink and ping that made me want to smile.

The noise that cut through was the sound Mam made and we all turned round with a jump. She fell hard on her knees on the doorstep as though someone had hit her from behind. The letter was clutched to her chest, open already, the envelope torn. Her eyes were shut tight but her mouth was wide open. My tummy turned cold inside and a bit slippery.

Mrs Kenny ran across the street from number 28, flour up to her elbows, arms outstretched to Mam. The motorbike man turned away as she reached her, kneeling beside her, wrapping Mam up. I wanted to go to her, but my legs weren't working. And I had to look after the motorbike.

Another door opened further up and Mrs Sankey came out, wiping her hands on her pinny as she crossed the road to Mam. Mrs Shelton next door but one stood on her doorstep, holding her hands like we did in church on Sundays, and it wasn't even the weekend.

The man walked back towards his bike. To me.

"Good job," he said as he got on again and I realised I was hardly breathing. "Sorry about your dad." He turned the key and kicked a pedal on the side. The engine started with a roar and I stumbled a step back.

"What's wrong with Dad?" I shouted over the noise.

He looked at me for a full second before he fitted his goggles back over his eyes.

"He's gone, lad," he said. The bike pulled away and I watched it all the way up Welbeck Street. The bounce of it over the cobbles. The occasional cough of exhaust.

And I thought, wherever Dad had gone, I hoped he'd gone on a motorbike.

I wasn't allowed out on the street for a few weeks after that. Mam kept me inside "where she could see me". Although sometimes she probably couldn't see me for all the other women who were there. The front room was always full, the kettle was always on. The door was always opening and shutting with Auntie Nellie or Auntie Biddy popping over to check on things. They weren't really my aunties, as Mam had no brothers or sisters of her own. She was like me.

An only child.

She kept telling the other women she was like her own mam too, Grandma Gates, who I'd never met but who apparently gave me my love of kippers.

"War widows, the pair of us, God bless her soul," Mam kept saying like she couldn't believe it. I didn't know what a widow was, but it was obviously not something she wanted to be.

"Just you and me now, Ernie," she'd say to me at night when she tucked me in and held me tight. I liked that bit, stuffed my face into her hair even though it tickled my nose. It didn't really feel much different to me at first, with Dad "gone", until I woke in the night and heard her crying in her bedroom. That gave me a pain in my tummy and I curled into a ball under the covers.

Every morning, she smiled at me when I came down but her eyes were red. I'd see her later in the kitchen with Auntie Bid, head in her hands at the table. Moments like that I wanted very much to stay inside, right next to her, but Auntie Bid decided it was time for me to start going out again.

"Don't need the boy to be hearing this," she said to Mam, pulling her own earlobe. I wondered if she was making fun of my ears, and felt my face get hot. Mam wiped her eyes and blinked as if she hadn't noticed me there. "Go find my Billy," Auntie Bid said to me and pointed at the front door. Then, miracle of miracles, she pulled a sweets ration slip from her purse, two whole ounces, and held it out to me.

"Tell Billy I said to share with you," she said and I didn't need telling twice. Mam even managed a watery smile and I was out the door before it got taken back.

While I was buying humbugs, the women made a plan.

By the time I'd sucked my tongue sore, it was sorted. Mam was working at the baker's and we'd live in the rooms above.

The Everyday

"We'll be in next, love," Phyllis said with a little pat on my hand.

"We've been waiting bloody long enough," I grumbled. The doctor's waiting room was full of infections and I didn't want her to catch anything. Nor me neither. I'd seen how quick a cold can turn into something much worse. The sooner we were out of there, the better.

Phyllis leaned forward and started rifling through the magazines on the table and I nudged her and shook my head. You couldn't see the little buggers, but there'd be germs all over the pages. She sighed and sat back, shaking her head with a little frown. A door opened and everyone looked towards it.

"Ernie Dawes."

I went to stand up, trying to use my thighs as leverage rather than touch the chair. But Phyl had to tuck one hand under my armpit and heave, and at last I was on my feet. Once we were inside the doctor's room, I felt a bit happier. I eased myself into a chair and loosened my coat.

"Nice to see you, Ernie," the doctor said. They get younger every day, I swear to God. Brown hair swept to the side, tanned face even in spring. I bet he was a jogger. One of those bouncing along the pavement in all weathers looking smug. He turned to his screen and I nodded in satisfaction when he at least had to put glasses on to read my notes. Not that young then. That made me feel better. At least he'd know what he was doing. Although I wasn't sure myself what we were doing. A check-up, Phyllis had said. Like an MOT for my bike. Now she put her bag at her feet and crossed her ankles.

"So…" the doctor said, twisting his chair back to me with a smile. "We're getting a bit forgetful, are we?"

"Eh?"

"Finding it hard to remember some things?" He tried again.

Bloody cheek. I folded my arms.

"It's not all the time, Doctor," Phyllis said. "Just sometimes." She patted my hand again and this time I held on. I didn't like the way he was looking at me.

"That's totally normal and it is part of ageing. So, in some ways, it's to be expected…" the doctor said, looking at his notes again, "…at your age, Ernie. Seventy-seven years young, eh?"

Patronising sod. I snorted. "Still working though, Doctor. Fit as a fiddle," I said with a little puff of my chest, and his eyebrows shot up his forehead at that.

"Just in the shop every now and then," Phyllis said. "High days and holidays really. He likes to help with the setting out. Makes the displays look nice for our Sue."

I did too. Nobody made the pyramids of grapefruit like I did. Or laid out the new fancy fruits, the kiwis and mangoes. I made them look like everyone should try them, not just the posh folk from Bell Ridge. Laid them in a little bit of straw, or on a palm leaf, it was all in the little things. Alf would have been proud of it. He'd taught me well.

"That's where I first noticed it," Phyllis said. "He couldn't remember some of the regulars' names. And then he started giving people the wrong change."

I kicked her foot. Why did she have to go and tell him that. Made me look right the fool.

Phyl smiled apologetically.

The doctor nodded, tapped his pen.

"Any other health problems?" he asked Phyllis, not me, so I stayed quiet. "Heart problems? Diabetes?"

She shook her head. "Never had a day's sick in his life, Doctor," she said.

He turned to me. I nodded my agreement. Healthy as a horse, me.

"Ernie, I want to ask you some questions," he said, coming round to my side of the desk and sitting on it.

He was a bit close now and my stomach was feeling a bit off, going round like a washing machine.

"What's your full name?" he said and I felt a little bubble of laughter inside. I knew that one.

"Ernie George Dawes."

"What's your date of birth?" he said next.

"Sixth February 1940," I said, pleased with myself now.

"Who is the prime minister?" he said then and that stopped me in my tracks. Was it that woman still? The one with the handbag? Or the fella with the big ears, like mine? I glanced at Phyllis but she didn't mouth me the answer. I glared at her.

"Margaret Thatcher," I said, hopefully. He wrote a little note on his pad and I knew I'd got it wrong. "Don't follow politics all that much," I said. "Load of talk and no action."

"And what year is it now?" the doctor said. I looked out the window, for a clue, but there was just a hazel tree, full of blue tits in and out of the branches.

"Ernie?" he said again and I set my brain to thinking. I felt about middle-aged. And I knew I'd been born at the start of the war, so that gave me a starter.

"1996?" I said and Phyllis gave my hand a little squeeze. I thought that meant I got it right but he wrote something on his pad again that told me different.

"Where did you grow up Ernie?"

I breathed a sigh of relief. Now I had it.

"Divine Street, Liverpool," I said. "Down by the docks. We were number 31. Never had an inside toilet. Just the one at the bottom of the garden. Then we moved above the baker's. My mam used to bring me little puffs of pastry that were too small for anything else at the end of her day. We called them butter bits." My mouth was literally watering at the memory. I grinned at Phyllis, pleased with myself.

"And what did you do yesterday?"

"Yesterday?"

What *had* I done yesterday?

My head wasn't helping. It felt black inside.

I could sense the doctor looking at me. I felt Phyllis rub my hand with her thumb.

"Not a lot," I said. "Just the usual."

"What was that then?" He wasn't letting me off, the sod. "Shopping? Gardening?"

Had I done those things? Suddenly unsure what to do or say, I glanced at Phyllis, just to see her there.

"Nothing really. Bit of a boring day!" I laughed it off.

The questions went on for hours it felt like. Where did I live? Who was in my family? What time was it? What month was it?

What day of the week was it? I mean! Who cares? They're all the same aren't they, without a working week to be done.

It got worse.

The doctor took a handful of coins out of his pocket and showed me them in his palm and asked me how much? My neck got hot and I wiped my fingers round my collar. He pointed at some things on the wall, a picture, a light, a round thing with numbers on it, for me to tell him what they were. He took my temperature, and held my wrist for a bit at one time, and I was pleased to put my hand back in Phyl's after. By the time he closed his pad and stood up, I felt a bit upset, like I'd got something wrong, but I didn't know what.

"You're right to bring him in, Mrs Dawes," the doctor said. "The cognitive assessment is pretty conclusive."

Phyllis shook her head as she tried to keep up with the words. I didn't even bother, just glad nobody was looking at me any more, waiting for me to make a fool of myself.

The blue tits I could see outside were back and forth between the hazel and the hedge, collecting little bits of twig and grass for nest building. They were a constant flash of blue and yellow and I wished I could hear them. I edged towards the window.

"The questions and answers we've just been through test out a whole range of things: short- and long-term memory, concentration span, orientation, for example his awareness of time and place."

I put my hands on the windowsill and noticed they shook a little.

"He remembers the past so well, though, Doctor. He's always talking about it," Phyllis said.

"It's common with dementia," the doctor said. "The far away replaces the everyday."

Two blue tits were fighting over a twig and didn't see a black cat prowling around the hedge line of the doctors' surgery. I banged on the window to startle the birds away to safety. It worked. The birds flew and the cat jumped, although so did Phyl and the doctor.

"I'm going to give you this leaflet to take away with you and read. It's a lot to take in." The doctor was back round his own side of the desk now, rummaging in his drawer and shuffling some papers together.

"I'm also going to book him in for some blood tests. Just to make sure there is nothing else going on. Maybe with his thyroid or his haemoglobin." His pen scratched at the paper pad. Good luck to someone reading that.

"But I'd like to see him again in a few months. Things can change very slowly with dementia, or sometimes overnight. And there'll be a time in the future when you might need a bit of help."

"Oh, we'll be fine," Phyllis said as she picked up her bag and shrugged herself back into her coat. It was the voice she'd use at the shop sometimes, the one that cheered people up if they were having a bad day. The "we're all in this together" kind of tone, normally accompanied by a free apple or banana and a hug. But it didn't make me feel any better today. She shouldn't have made me come here. I didn't like it.

When we were outside, I let her have it.

"Made me look right daft," I muttered. "All those stupid questions."

Phyllis took the car keys out of her bag and set off across the tarmac.

"Just cos I can't remember the Queen's birthday!" I snorted, letting her lead the way.

"I mean, what if my brain is going to mush?" I was cross now. Felt like I'd been bullied. Like when the boys at school used to make fun of my ears, running round the yard calling me Lugs or Wing Nut. She was still a step ahead of me, like she was in a rush.

"What if it really *is* going to mush? Like a mouldy cabbage? You going to throw me on the compost heap?"

She turned round then, and I felt even worse because she was crying. Just a bit and quietly. But enough to make me hate myself.

"Never," she said. "You might be an old fool. But you're *my* old fool." And she gave me a hug right there in the car park.

Then I felt better.

Nina

"Nina – you're wearing the floor out," Sue said and put a hand out to stop her daughter on the next circuit of the shop. Nina had popped in to see her on the way home from college and had been circling the island in the middle of the shop for the past fifteen minutes. It was piled high with fruit and vegetables in every size, shape and colour you could wish for. If you liked fruit and vegetables that is. Nina didn't much. She'd rather have a Big Mac and chips any day of the week, but Mum had decided that fast food might be making her concentration worse. But just the thought of salty fries made her mouth water. She wondered how much money she had in her account and whether she could sneak a sly burger in lunch at college now and again.

"Make yourself useful." Mum pointed at a freshly delivered crate of pomegranates by the back door.

"I was going to go home," Nina said. "I've got homework to do."

"First I've heard of it," Sue said and nodded at the fruit again.

Nina clenched her teeth together to stop anything nasty coming out and dragged the crate across the shop's floor.

It might be the first her mum had heard of it, but it was true. In fact, Nina had so much homework she didn't know where to start. She'd begun a few of the assignments, several times, and now had different drafts in different folders and none of them finished. Others she hadn't started yet. She'd got as far as reading the titles, or maybe even opening a new Word document, but then something else had happened, or a song had come on that she liked, and she'd sung, or she'd danced, or she'd remembered she had to water the plants on her bedroom window. She really liked them there, lining the sill, but, by the time she'd watered them and pruned any dead leaves and tucked in any protruding roots, she'd forgotten about whichever assignment she was thinking of working on. She knew there were more assignments too. Ones that she hadn't even looked at yet. Waiting there. Hanging in the Teams conversations with her various tutors. Again she wished she'd picked other subjects. The ones she'd chosen really sucked. She attacked the pomegranate crate with scissors to open it up as her mum was serving a couple of women, both with buggies in tow.

Geography. Nina had honestly thought it would be field trips and conservation. She liked animals, kind of. Although thinking about it, she probably preferred plants. But the topics so far this term had been about urbanisation and how to decrease traffic flow in big cities and she really didn't care about car sharing or congestion charging or staggered working hours. The first layer of pomegranates was red and shiny. She arranged them in neat rows, one on top of the other, until they were symmetrically beautiful.

English literature. She was halfway through *Tess of the D'Urbervilles* but she'd read the last page already to see how it ended. She'd gone online to read reviews as well to see if she could get a few spoilers of the story, but then found one reviewer called "Ihatebooks" who gave it a one-star review for being "too old". She thought that was hilarious and then ended up reading every other review that "Ihatebooks" had ever written. *The Catcher in the Rye* – too American. *Pride and Prejudice* – too snobby. She lost all track of time and what page she was on and she'd never got back to it since. She'd lined up half of the fruit now, it looked glossy in the fake straw of the display.

Sport. She liked running. Or jumping. Or hitting balls. That made everything inside her quieten down for that moment. It was about being absorbed. Like when she did a puzzle or constructed something with Lego. That made everything calm too. She could just focus on the puzzle pieces and how they fit together. Mum had laughed at her when she told her how good it felt to put things together and said that as far as she knew there were no professional puzzler jobs available, so perhaps she should instead get on with her sport homework.

But the homework stayed undone because it made her feel fizzy inside just to look at it. Pages of text to read. Workbooks to go through. Diagrams of muscles and bones to label. It all remained blank.

Now the pomegranates were all out, she could smell their smell. If she had to pick one fruit she liked, it would probably be pomegranates. Not because of the taste, but because of how she ate them. She used a pin to pick out each tiny pink segment individually, and it took her hours and hours and kept her fingers busy.

"Thanks love, that looks great," Sue said when the women left the shop, their purchases in paper bags in the trays at the bottoms of the buggies. A tiny treat having been given for the babies, a strawberry each, as they left. A tradition that Pops had started when he opened the shop, said it came from the stall with Grandad Alf long before that. Give the little ones a piece of fruit for free and the mothers will come back.

"How was college today, then?" Her mum had a special look when she asked this question every day. It was almost like she was dreading the answer.

"Fine," Nina lied.

Her mum peered at her and asked her usual next question.

"Get any marks back?"

Nina shook her head.

"Not yet." And she wouldn't do any time soon, because she hadn't yet handed in any work to get marked. Her foot started to tap to try to get rid of the bad feeling in her stomach.

"Meet any new people?" Mum looked hopeful now and this was the face Nina hated the most. She knew Sue wanted her to be like Jessica and Josh. Meeting new people every week. Going to the parties and the pub and the places to be. But she wasn't like them. She could only be like herself.

"Actually, I did meet some new people today," she heard herself saying and Sue's face relaxed. Nina couldn't help but smile, think how easy it was to make her mother happy. And it wasn't exactly a lie. "In the canteen." She bent to pick up the crate so that she could look at something else.

"That's great, love. Remember, it's only been a term. These things take time."

Nina had met new people in the canteen that day. That was true. But she didn't think they'd be hanging out with her any time soon. She'd been sitting on her own and eating her sandwiches, watching the groups of girls and boys sitting on tables, grouped around bags, throwing crisps at each other. A couple of them glanced over at her every now and then, or talked behind their hands, but nobody called her over or waved.

She'd put her earphones in and ignored them as best she could. After that, they'd been oblivious to her altogether. Until, that was, a few minutes later when she was watching a plane cross the sky outside the common room window leaving a vapour trail behind it. She'd been wondering about the people on the plane and where they might be going and if they might be eating one of those lunches that comes on a little plastic tray, because she'd love to do that. Then a little brown bird landed right there on the windowsill and looked in the glass at her. Literally, only a few feet away, she couldn't stop staring at it. The tiny little matchstick legs and the beady little eyes. It puffed up its feathers in the breeze, but kept staring at her. Then it turned and darted away and, as it did, she laughed out loud and called to it, "Fly away birdie!" But because she had her headphones on, it must have come out louder than she meant, because when she looked round everyone within ten tables' vicinity was staring at her.

And then they laughed. In fact, they roared as they fell about laughing and flapping their arms like wings. Since then, everywhere she went, she heard people tweeting behind her in the corridors and she knew that word had spread. She would now officially be known at college as "Birdie", Nina was sure.

Sue was still staring at Nina as though she wanted to ask something else, but the shop bell jingled again and saved her.

Nan came in first while Pops shuffled in behind. Sue came out from behind the counter to greet them with kisses for Nan and hugs for Pops. Nina came close afterwards and did the same.

"There's my TillyMint," Pops said as she squeezed him. His breath smelled of mint humbugs so Nina knew they must have been somewhere in the car, as they kept a stash in the glove compartment. He used to let her have one from the tin when he picked her up after school sometimes.

"Want a cuppa?" her mum asked, nodding towards the kettle out the back, but Nan shook her head.

"We won't stay," she said. "Just passing on the way home from the doctors."

"How did it go?" Sue asked and her face had the same look it had recently when she asked Nina about college.

"Big fat waste of time," Pops snorted and set off towards the cabbage corner to inspect the produce. He couldn't resist rearranging them.

Nan waited till he was absorbed and then stage-whispered to her daughter, "As we thought. Dementia. He'll need more tests to determine what type, but it's definite."

Nina drummed her fingers on the box of pomegranates.

"What does it actually mean though?" Sue asked, watching Pops as though expecting him to suddenly do something unusual. But he was just arranging cabbages into a perfect pyramid, standard practice for him. Nan pulled a leaflet out of her bag and pushed it over the counter. Nina thought Nan looked like she'd been crying.

"It's more than just forgetting the odd thing," she said. "In the end you forget everything. The people you knew. How to walk. How to talk. How to eat." Nan got a tissue out of her bag and blew her nose, and Sue moved round the counter to be closer.

"You sure you won't stay for a tea?" she said as if that would solve everything.

Nina felt the fizz growing inside her. She stood on one foot, then the other. Then she hopped up the aisle to her pops, who was close to completing a pyramid of cabbages.

"Cabbage-tastic," Nina told him and he nodded. He had a cap on his head that made his ears look all the bigger. He used to waggle them when she was young and pretend to take off, like Dumbo.

"You working today?" he asked.

Nina shook her head, wishing it actually was a Saturday. "Nope, college today, Pops."

He picked up an apple from the display and buffed it against his sleeve before tossing it towards her. She caught it and he grinned, like she'd done something good, and it made her feel better inside. She didn't want to think of her pops not being Pops. She didn't want to think he might not remember all the good things he'd done for her, with her. It was he who had bought the trampoline for her birthday and surprised her with it, after constructing it overnight in the back garden with her dad. "For when the fizzing gets a bit much," he'd said to her quietly. They'd had to buy two more since then – they certainly got a lot of use.

"Classes going any better?"

"Not really." Nina turned the apple round in her hand, selecting her first bite. "Not sure I'm cut out for college." She bit cleanly and the juice spurted into her mouth.

Pops shrugged as if it really didn't matter. Like it wouldn't ruin her life or whatever Mum thought would happen.

"You just need to find your passion," he said.

"Like your motorbike," she said round a mouthful of apple, before he did.

"Exactly," he said. Nina wished it was that simple. Maybe things had been easier in the olden days. What had Pops ever had to worry about apart from running the shop? Things were more complicated now.

She watched him as he straightened up a few sticks of rhubarb and then picked off a few wrinkled grapes as they passed back down the aisle. He pointed at the onion section and said, exactly as she knew he would, "That's shallot of onions!" before chuckling at his own joke.

He stopped at the bananas, close to the cash desk where Nan and Mum were talking loudly about the weather and what they might have for tea as though they hadn't been discussing his health at all.

"My mum used to love bananas," Pops said suddenly, holding a bunch in his hand and staring at it as though seeing something else entirely. "She'd be your great-grandmother – Josephine," he said to Nina, who knew that much already. She'd done a family tree project at primary. Pops had helped her with it. Told her at the time he was lucky to have a family at all. It had been a close thing apparently.

"You couldn't get them in the war and she had to wait years to have a banana again. Can you imagine that, TillyMint?" He gave her a nudge in the ribs with his elbow to make his point, and Nina heard her nan stage-whisper again, "Listen to him! You really wouldn't think there was anything wrong with that memory at all, would you?"

The Far Away

1945

The next time a motorbike stopped at our house, it brought Alf on it. Mam's new friend.

It was a Sunday, the bakery was closed and Mam had slept in until nine, instead of having to get up and shape the loaves first thing. Sundays were the best day of the week according to Mam and that morning she sang to the wireless and told me we'd have a guest for tea.

It was the way she said it that made it important. That, and the fact she made me wash my face twice. People came round all the time, Auntie Nell, Mrs Peters, or Billy's mum, but Mam never announced them in advance. Since Dad had been gone, the women just turned up with a call as they came up the stairs and Mam would put the kettle on. Sometimes they'd bring a pinch of tea with them and other times they'd drink ours. It felt to me as if one or other of them were always around, talking, sewing, laughing. They'd pinch my cheeks and be kind about my ears, and the whole flat seemed fuller with them in it.

But this time, Mam had made an afternoon tea, with tongue in the sandwiches and a whole scone each from the shop. She'd saved our jam for weeks to dollop on top. I knew it was a special occasion. I hadn't seen her so excited since VE Day, when she'd danced in the street and thrown her hat in the air.

Her new friend had apparently been in and out of the baker's every day for a month just so that he could talk to her. He said her smile was worth walking the mile from the docks. After that he took her to the pictures once or twice and to a dance hall that had opened on Walker Street. I stayed at Billy Sankey's then, back on Divine Street, which was fine but we had to share his bed and he kicked like a donkey. I preferred my own bed.

Mam heard the motorbike engine in the road outside at the same time as me and rushed to the mirror to pinch her cheeks to give her a bit of colour. I pressed my nose flat to the window as he pulled up and Mam flashed me a smile as she ran to the stairs to let him in.

My breath steamed up the glass and I wiped it clear. His motorbike was army green and rattled as he turned it off. I wondered if it had been used in the war, across battlefields and to the Front. I saw him walk towards the shop door and then lost him from view.

When Mam brought her new fella up the stairs, I was stunned by the size of him. Alf had a big red nose and hands as wide as a ham hanging in the butcher's window. They grabbed at Mam and lifted her clean off the ground as he danced her in a little jig to the music playing on the wireless. They pulled her to him and she looked tiny against his chest, as if he could smother her completely in his coat if he wanted to, pulling the two sides together and hiding her, then opening it again like a magic trick. She came away breathless and smiling.

"Get away with you," she said, but it didn't sound like she meant it one bit. I suddenly wanted to be closer to her, so that I could hold on and she would look at me instead. My shuffling caught her attention and she smoothed her hair back off her forehead and calmed herself.

She reached out her hand to me.

"This is Ernie," she said, and I slipped my hand into hers.

His head swung in my direction and I felt my ears getting hot. They always seemed to be the first thing people saw about me. His eyes were surprisingly blue under eyebrows black as coal. I held my breath.

"Ah, the man of the house," he said and stuck his hand out towards me.

Mam nudged me gently with an elbow and I stumbled a step towards him. My hand disappeared into his palm, and he shook my hand like he was pumping the water tap on the corner.

"Nice to meet you, Ernie."

His eyes had deep lines from the corners, crinkling white in his face. They reminded me of seagulls' wings. Mam had told me he used to be a merchant seaman.

"Nice to meet you too, Mister," I repeated, not quite sure what to call him and hoping my arm wouldn't come out of its socket. He stopped shaking then and glanced back at Mam.

"I wanted to bring you some sweets," he said and I sucked in my breath in anticipation. "But there was nothing doing. Nobody had any coupons to swap this week."

I let my breath out slowly at the loss. Nobody ever gave us anything like presents, mainly because nobody had anything to give. We traded and borrowed, and lent if we had it. "We were all in the same boat," Mam said.

All through the war, Mam lent Mrs Green half a crown on a Friday to see her through the weekend and then Mrs Green gave it back on a Monday when she got her wages. That went on for so long that when Mrs Green finally went off to live with her sister in Manchester they couldn't remember whose half a crown it was. So they split it down the middle and hugged goodbye. Everyone was the same, give it if you've got it, take it back when you need. Apart from mean old Mr Brent. He got free coal from working at the yard and still took Mam's butter allowance off her if she ever needed a bucketful. That was so mean, and Mam let me spit on the pat before we passed it over.

Alf grinned at Mam now like they had a secret. But then he said he had something even better for me and my hands pressed themselves into little fists of excitement. What could be better than a sweet? He put his hand in the pocket of his great black overcoat and then pulled out something the length of his hand and yellow. Black stripes on its sides. It curved like a smile. I'd never seen anything like it before in my life.

"This is a banana," he said, and Mam clapped her hands to the sides of her face.

"Where did you manage to get hold of that?" she asked but he just winked in reply and tapped a finger the size of a sausage to the side of his conk.

"It's for you." He held it towards me.

"Lucky you, Ernie," Mam said as I took it in my hand. It felt soft and hard at the same time. "Haven't had one of those since before the war. They are so delicious!"

I examined it. The skin was smooth and my nail left a crescent in it when I pressed. One end had a tint of green to it, the other ended in a bit that looked like wood. I smelled it but it smelled like nothing. They were both watching me so I bit into it.

Alf roared. Head back, mouth like a red tunnel, something boggling about down his throat.

"No, love," rushed Mam, pulling it away from my mouth. "You've got to peel it first."

I wiped my mouth on the back of my hand – disgusting. The peel had squeaked against my teeth.

Mam showed me how to snap the top back and then pull the skin down. She did one side and then let me do the rest until the yellow flaps hung over my hand and the naked banana curved towards my mouth. I didn't like the cold limpness of the banana's skin against my own.

"There you go, son," Mam said and licked her own lips.

I took a bite, more cautious this time. Chewed carefully, felt the banana mush in my mouth.

"What do you think of that, eh?" Alf asked, as though he already knew the answer.

I swallowed. Scratched my tongue against my front teeth. They felt coated, slimy. "I'd rather have a lollipop," I said.

Alf bellowed, head back, stomach jiggling.

"Ernie!" Mam rolled her eyes.

"He'd rather have a lollipop," he spluttered to Mam and then turned to me. "I'll remember that next time." Alf ruffled my hair before holding his hand out for the banana, which I was glad to pass over. He presented it to Mam with a bow. I've never seen her eat anything so fast in my life.

Mam let him sit in Dad's seat by the fire. We all still called it Dad's seat even though I couldn't remember him sitting in it. Maybe if I closed my eyes tight I could recall his knees as he rested there. Me holding on to them as I balanced. If I focused really hard, I could almost hear him laughing at me. "Go on, lad, that's the way." But maybe I was just making that up.

Alf made Dad's chair look small. His knees were bent and came up high, and his arms hung off the sides. But he settled back into it and made it look like the most comfortable seat in the world. Mam beamed at him and put the kettle on.

And after that, it was Alf's seat.

He came every Sunday. Always with a different surprise for Mam or for me. The first week after I met him, a sugar cane, which turned my lips pink as I sucked. The second week, two mackerel, wrapped in newspaper, which made Mam clap her hands. After that, some herring, which made me burp, then a jar of liquor that made Mam hiccup and, finally, some nylons that made her shake her head in wonder. He was like a magician, I thought. Or "a chancer," I heard Mrs Green say to Mam. Or "too good to be true to look at me when I've got Ernie too," said Mam, at which point Mrs Green seemed to agree with her.

But whatever he was, it got to the point that we heard the motorbike and both of us would smile and run to the stairs.

"Is it fast?" I asked him, standing beside the bike one Sunday when he arrived.

"Faster than you've ever been," he said, unclipping his helmet.

"What's it feel like?" I asked him.

"Like freedom," he said. "That's why I call her Libby. Short for Liberty."

I thought about that feeling for a moment trying to imagine it. I could only think of the time Billy and I went down the hill on a go-kart when Mam wasn't watching.

"Do all bikes have names?" I asked and, when he nodded a yes, I asked Mam what her name was short for.

The Everyday and Far Away

"Josie is short for Josephine," she said with a smile.

"I'm going to get one when I'm older," I said, never surer of anything in my life. "And when I do, I'm going to call her Josephine."

"Then we can ride together," Alf said and Mam dropped her eyes and blushed, before she lifted them to him again.

He plonked the helmet on my head, and did it up beneath my chin. My ears were squished against the sides, sticking out like they did, but it was a small price to pay as then he did what I'd wanted him to do since the first day. He lifted me under the arms and sat me on the saddle.

"Careful, Ernie," Mam said, like something could happen me just sitting on it. She was always like that, maybe more so since Dad was gone.

"The boy's grand," Alf said and took his hands off me, rather suddenly. I clamped my knees to the side of the saddle for balance and reached forward for the handlebars but they were too far away. The bike wobbled very slightly on its stand and my knees pinned themselves to the tank. I shuffled forward on the seat until I was almost lying horizontal but had the handgrips in my fingers. Mam laughed and Alf put his arm round her shoulders. The bike had a smell to it, oil and rain and wet metal.

"Vroom, vroom," I said, moving my hand on the grip. The helmet slid slowly down my forehead until it covered my eyes and I heard the sound of a kiss before Mam lifted it back up and unfastened it.

"Come on, you," she said. "Off."

I slipped off to one side, but let my fingers run along the tank as I was led away.

Every weekend after that, Alf asked me if I wanted to clean the motorbike, and off I'd go with a bucket of water and an old rag from under the sink.

"It will take you at least an hour to do a good job," he'd say to me and wink at Mam. "We'll be down to inspect when you're done. So no rush, eh? I'm counting on you."

I was so proud of that job, people stopping to look at her on the street. And when Alf did come down, he was always in a good mood, pleased with my efforts. He'd have time to chat and show me things about Libby.

"This is the fuel tank, and every now and then you have to clean it out. Flush it through to make sure everything runs smoothly.

"These are the panniers. It's a posh word for saddlebags. I keep my treasures in there.

"This is the exhaust pipe. People stick potatoes in them sometimes for the laugh. They make a big bang when you start up. So, it's a good idea to check for a potato before you get on.

"This mirror shows you what's going on behind you. You always want to know that, Ernie, believe me."

Sometimes he'd even take bits off the bike to show me how they went back on. I could have done it all day long, but he always wanted to get back to Mam. And she didn't even really like bikes. He was hard to understand like that.

It got to the point that the weekdays seemed quiet compared to when Alf was there. He arrived with a roar, pulled something precious from his panniers, and presented it to Mam with an "ask no questions" tap of his nose. And Mam didn't really want to know where his gifts came from. All she knew was that her widow's pension could never afford the things he bought. So she'd pocket his offerings with a soft smile.

Upstairs, Alf took up so much space that we had to edge around each other to get to the stove, or down the stairs for the loo. His boots were longer than the loaf tins and he had to duck his head to come in the doorway. But I liked him there, slapping his thigh when he laughed.

Mam liked it too. I could tell. It wasn't like she was sad in the week, but she was definitely happier at the weekend. All week long she rose early to shape the loaves before helping to stack them in the oven even though she was meant to work at the counter. But it was a deal she'd come to, with the baker. If she helped with the early shift, she could use the oven after the day's baking was finished. Its heat was still enough to cook a casserole or a stew, and this saved our gas, she told me. So every morning, often before it got light, she'd leave the door on the latch and head downstairs. Then she'd pop up to me to make a bit of toast for breakfast and get me off to school before tucking her hair under her headscarf for the shop. After school, I'd play outside for a bit while she practised her icing for the wedding cakes with a piping bag and some mashed potato. Sopping up our casserole with a bread roll and some margarine, we'd listen to the wireless in the evenings. She'd pull out my bed in the living room by eight and take herself off to the tiny bedroom to read, turning the lamp out by nine so that she could get up for the early bread the next morning. It was just us, and we were used to the way it was.

But now Mam was like a movie star on a Sunday. She curled her hair, wearing it in white rags all Saturday night to be bouncy in the morning. And she fluttered about Alf, touching his forearm with her fingertips and turning her face up to smile. Sometimes they seemed to forget I was in the room, their faces turned to each other, their voices low. Then I'd shuffle and cough and Alf would nudge me with his elbow, fair knocking me off my feet.

"You're keeping us in line, eh, Ernie?"

"He's a good boy," Mam said to Alf, as though to reassure him. "Never any trouble."

"Must be about time for the bike to get its clean," Alf would suggest and I didn't need asking twice. I'd be happy to leave them on their own for a bit of kissing and making eyes, if it meant I got time with the motorbike.

I was out there one time, rubbing and buffing, when George Malone came round the corner with his brother. He didn't like me much, ever since I told Mam he pushed me over and she told his mum to sort him out.

"Polishing your mam's fancy man's bike again?"

I didn't know what a fancy man was but it didn't sound nice. I kept my head down and hoped he'd go away but my guts were churning.

"Don't blame him not wanting you around," he sneered. "Snot nose." I heard him sniff.

"Getting in the way," he said. "My dad said no bloke wants some other fella's kid" – and he hawked up and spat. A shiny silver glob landed on the front wheel arch. "Specially one with ears like yours."

"Don't do that," I said, horrified, not by what he said, but what he'd done.

"Make me!" He kicked me hard in the backside as I leaned forward to clean off the spit.

The Everyday and Far Away

I grunted and squinted my eyes tight shut. My eyes were burning and I bit my lip hard to stop any crying coming out. Using the corner of my cloth, I dipped it in the water and rubbed the arch clean.

"Mummy's boy," he said as he walked away and I waited till I couldn't hear his footsteps any more before I wiped my eyes.

"Don't let him do that again," Alf said suddenly, stepping out from the doorway. I felt my face go red in shame. He'd not let me look after his bike again if I let someone gob on it.

"I've cleaned it off, Alf," I said, pointing a shaking finger towards the wheel. Alf followed my finger with his eyes, frowned and then shook his head.

"No," he said. "I mean, don't let him do that again *to you*."

The kick. He'd seen the kick.

"He's always a bit handy," I said, trying to shrug it off but knowing I wouldn't sit down properly till the weekend.

"He's not just mean with his hands. He's mean with his mouth. Don't let him talk to you like that again."

I looked at him. What was I supposed to do if George Malone wanted to say things to me? He was bigger than me, and older. And everyone in the street was scared of him.

"Next time, wallop him one," Alf said, putting both hands up in front of his chest like a boxer.

"Mam would kill me," I said automatically, thinking how she always said to walk away if there was any trouble.

"She doesn't need to know," he said. "This is men's stuff."

I considered that for a moment, then put my hands up in front of me, like his.

Alf smiled and nodded.

"That's the way, Ernie. I can show you how. We'll not have anyone talking to you like that again, eh, lad?" He looked up at the window to see if Mam was watching. "Not here though, eh?" He nodded his head towards the passage and I followed with just a quick look over my shoulder.

There in the backyard, he held his palms towards me at my shoulder height and told me to hit them. He showed me how to curl my fists properly with my thumb flat on top and then told me to hit his great flat hands, one after the other until my arms felt like they might fall out of their sockets. Then he took me in the bakery store and set me against a sack of flour, the scratchy material shredding my knuckles until they bled. All good for the hardening, Alf said. He taught me a one-two, an uppercut and a sidie. And all the time he encouraged me along with the thought of George Malone's face.

"Here he is, Ernie…"

"He just called you a mummy's boy, Ernie…"

"What you got for Georgie boy today, Ernie?"

"That's the last time he'll spit on a motorbike, lad!"

And it was the spit I saw, rather than George's face. Then I punched harder and grunted with the effort of each and every swing.

"Good lad," Alf said at last when my breath heaved and huffed out of my chest like a steam train.

"Practise those moves, Ernie, and use 'em when you need 'em."

I smiled. I'd not let anything happen to the bike again.

I never saw Alf treat Libby so rough as he did the day he rode away. He usually stroked her side or patted her saddle with a gentle hand. But that day, he kicked the stand so hard it made me wince, it must have left a dent. He flung his leg over and sat down in one move, and the bike groaned down on what it had left of its suspension. He pulled his helmet on without looking back up at the window at Mam like he always did and put his goggles over eyebrows that almost hid his eyes.

It was like he was already somewhere else in his head. He didn't seem to see me on the kerb. Normally, he'd give me a salute or a wink as he went. But not that day. It made me half want to step forward, and half want to slink out of sight. He kicked the starter, once, twice, with no response. Swore something special under his breath and kicked it again before it roared into life.

Every other kid in the street turned to look, he revved it so much before he pulled away. And then he was gone. Up the high street and left into the square. Gone.

Something caught my eye and I saw it was Mam in the window. She had one hand against the glass and the other pressed to her chest. I turned away quick, not wanting her to see me.

The look on her face took me back to the early days without Dad. When she used to cry after putting me to bed. Or pick at her nails until they bled. I stayed out till the street lights came on, but something didn't feel right in my chest and I had to go home eventually. I dragged my feet on the stairs, not wanting to see Mam's face. I just knew something was wrong.

And as I opened the door to the rooms, I heard Auntie Nellie's voice and let out a sigh of relief that it wouldn't just be me. I'd got used to it being more than just me and Mam, and her sad. It had felt good to have Alf in our house, on our side. I'd got used to the sudden rumble of his laugh. The hair on the backs of his hands.

The smell of the sea on him as he came in the door. He made us stronger somehow. He made us a gang.

"Shhh pet," Aunt Nell was saying, like she might do to one of the babies. "No point crying."

"Gone and blown it, though, haven't I?"

I sat down on the top step, kept the door just ajar, knowing if I went in they'd change the subject.

"What exactly did you say?"

"I told him we'd better tie the knot, what with the bun in the oven."

"And? How'd he take it?"

"He said, if we tie the knot, we lose my widow's pension."

"He's got a point."

"But it's only a few shillings. Hardly worth the weight in my purse."

"But the docks are laying off, Josie. Maybe he's worried."

"And then I got to thinking. Maybe that's not the only reason."

"You've lost me, pet. You know he's mad about you."

"It's not just me he's getting, though is it? That's the point."

I could hear one of them moving about, and a glass clink on the table. Drinks were poured.

"Well, you can't do anything about that, love, can you?"

"Properly messed it up though, Nell," Mam said and this time her voice sounded like she was choking. "I don't think he's coming back," she said and then it sounded like she started crying and I creaked the door closed again and sat on the stairs till it stopped.

There was a quiet about the next few days. I hadn't realised how much noise Alf made until he wasn't there. Now my footsteps echoed as I ran across the room in the night to the potty and sometimes I could hear Mam crying into her pillow at night as though she were laying right next to me.

But we carried on as usual. The loaves were shaped in the mornings and the smell of dough woke me. School still expected me to be there, although my mind wasn't on it. Never the brightest in class, I was now the dud for a while, dragging my brain through reading and writing when it couldn't think straight. I played out after school each day, running with Billy and the dog, who was teasing Milly Wainright for having teeth that knocked on the door before she came round the corner. But that didn't really make me laugh. I had a big stone in my throat that threatened to stop my voice coming out or make me cry and I never knew which one it might be.

Mam took to calling me in, something she hadn't done for months. She'd appear in the baker's door, and pause, looking up to the square and all the other way to the corner, before she called me. I knew she was looking for Alf.

I wasn't looking for him. I was *listening* for him. My ears were perfect for the job, the size they were, and they felt like they were constantly turned on, they twitched like antennae. The occasional engine in the distance made me stop my game, skid to a halt until I recognised it was the enclosed sound of a car rather than the rev of the bike. It was never him.

Evenings were endless. Mam knitted. She was making a blanket, she said. But it didn't look big enough to me. Every now and then she'd stop and rub her eyes, like they were sore, or wet.

I drew pictures and organised my cigarette cards, identifying any for swapping and keeping my best in the box beside my bed.

But mostly I just shuffled them from hand to hand. I squeezed her extra tight at night, wanting her to smile at me right up to her eyes. She tried really hard, but it didn't quite make it. There was a weight on her. On me. In the air. It felt like we were both waiting. For him to come back. Or for him to be gone. Properly.

It was a Saturday I heard his bike again. I was crouched on the kerb, playing jacks with Billy. Libby. I'd know the rev and the slight rattle anywhere. The lump in my throat suddenly got so big I couldn't swallow.

I pushed myself to my feet, ignoring Billy's moans about it being his turn as I imagined the bike moving through the streets, coming closer. It was another few seconds before it turned in at the end of our street and sputtered slowly down the middle of the cobbles, minding the kids and the dog. I was right. It was him. I pressed my lips together, not sure what I wanted to say.

I stood there, legs not working enough to move, and he pulled to the kerb next to me, but as he took his helmet off I dropped my eyes. I didn't want to see his face in case it was bad news.

"Where's your mam?"

I pointed at the shop. Where else would she be on a Saturday?

"You coming, Ernie?" he asked and turned towards the bakery. There was a queue out the door and he just excused himself all the way past them.

"Sorry ladies, only a minute. Just need a word with Josie there."

There were a few tuts but more cocked eyebrows and strained necks as they watched him go by. I followed, not wanting to be left behind.

Mam looked up from serving an old fella with his loaf as we walked in. When she saw Alf, her eyes widened and she clamped her teeth onto her bottom lip.

"You don't mind me butting in, do you? I just need to talk to Josie for a minute," he said to the next woman in the queue and she shook her head, looked like she was settling in to watch a show. Mam wiped her hands on her apron and then clasped them across her tummy. I'd seen her doing that a lot lately.

"Who else does the cakes, Josie?" Alf asked across the counter.

Mam looked at him as if he was speaking a different language. The line of women stopped their chattering, all the better to hear.

"The wedding cakes you mix and make? The ones you ice for practice with the mashed potato?"

"Why?" Mam asked.

"Cos you can't be making your own wedding cake, can you? That wouldn't be right at all."

He put his hand over the counter to her and she looked him right in the face before she put hers in it. She let him lead her out so that she was the customer side with him, while all the women in the shop craned their necks and the ones outside shuffled round the window to get a better view. And right then and there, Alf lowered himself onto one knee on the bakery floor and pulled out a little ring from the inside pocket of his overcoat.

Mam was only just taller than him still, even with him kneeling, and she put one hand to her chest, and the other on her belly, and smiled so all her teeth showed and her eyes went shiny.

"Josephine Dawes, will you marry me?" Alf said, holding the ring out towards her.

I realised I was holding my breath, watching Mam's face, and I wasn't the only one. I swear I could hear Mrs Greaves's tummy rumble next to me.

"Course I will," Mam said and the whole queue laughed and clapped while Alf pushed the ring onto her finger. When he lumbered back up to his feet and covered her up in a hug and a kiss it made the little line cheer, and someone said, "That's got to be worth a free loaf to celebrate, eh, Mr James?" And then everyone laughed at the baker's face.

"What about the widow's pension?" Mam said.

"You're worth more than money, my girl," Alf said, and I felt a bit dizzy.

He was staying.

When Mam came out of the kiss, her cheeks were so red it looked like she'd just done the kneading. She saw me there behind Alf and put a hand out towards me. I was pulled into their hug and it smelled like sea air and dough.

And after that Libby was always parked outside our house.

The Everyday

The little hand in mine was tugging me along, "C'mon GrandPops…" she lisped from a mouth more gap than teeth.

"Where to?" I asked but she just laughed and rolled her eyes, pulling again on my fingers.

I smiled at her. She was a determined little thing, Daisy, my great-granddaughter. She knew exactly what she wanted and precisely when she wanted it. And right now, she wanted me to go to the stream running at the bottom of the recreation field. "To see if fish go to sleep at night."

Phyllis and the others were waiting by the bonfire. There were going to be fireworks later apparently. They were all there. The whole family. Who would have thought I'd end up with one as big as that. When I came from such a small one in the first place.

Phyllis peered into the dark until she spotted me, then waved her gloved hand to make sure I'd seen her as I got pulled towards the water. She always liked to know where I was these days, it seemed. Like she was worried I was going to get lost. As if… We'd lived round here fifty years. I waved back with my free hand, shuffling behind my pint-sized guide down the slope to the sandy bank. The stream was ahead, clean and shallow, bubbling over a stony bottom. And probably bloody freezing. We stood side by side on the bank, a safe distance from the edge, to look.

"Maybe they are in their beds," Daisy announced. I didn't know who she was talking about but she was on to the next thing.

She let go of my hand, picked up a stick from the ground, and threw it into the stream and shouted, "splash."

"Shoes off!" I ordered and she looked at me in surprise. Her mouth a perfect little o. But then when she saw I was serious, and we were going to go paddling in the dark and in the winter, she threw herself onto the floor and yanked at her purple wellies. I knew if I sat down that far I'd never get back up, so I leaned against the willow trunk and bent slowly towards my feet. Daisy was already digging her toes into the cold wet sand and squirming in delight. She lifted a handful and let it run through her fingers.

"Come ONNNNNNNNN GrandPops!" she said again and I pointed at my bare feet, proud I'd managed to push my shoes and socks off, however awkwardly.

"Your trousers are gonna get wet," she said, pointing back and then launching herself at my shins. "You need to roll them up…"

She grunted with concentration, fingers pulling at the hem of my trousers. Chinos, Phyllis called them.

"Ta-da!" She bounced up and down in front of me and I saw she'd half-pushed and half-rolled my trousers up to my kneecap. Two white old hairy legs stuck out the bottom. They didn't look much like mine but I guessed they were.

"Good job, Daise," I said and she saluted me, just like I'd taught her. Made me smile every time.

"Right…" I said, trying to summon my courage to step into the water. She didn't hesitate, ran straight in, shrieked like she was dying and ran straight out again.

"BRRRRRRRR," she said and shook herself like a dog. I put out my hand and she slipped hers in.

The Everyday and Far Away

"Ready?" I said and we stepped in together, little and large. Big and dinky.

Just like Dinky Dot.

Mam had carried the baby into the house, my sister, wrapped in a white blanket so that only her face showed. It was red and screwed up, like she was determined to keep her eyes shut, no matter what happened. Alf came in behind them, carrying Mam's bag, smiling from one side of his face to the other.

Mam pulled me into her spare arm, close against her chest, and I felt her mouth on the back of my head, dropping kisses to make up for the ones I'd missed while she'd been away. It had only been a week but I'd never been without her before. My tummy felt better to have her back.

"Here she is," she said and carefully moved the blanket away from the squally-looking face. "This is Dot."

I tried not to breathe on her in case I woke her up. Alf fair beamed as he sat next to us in the chair.

"She's so tiny," I said, plucking up the courage to touch her cheek with a finger that shook. I knew how important she was. I'd heard Mam saying to Alf one night at the fire that the baby made the family complete. This was how it was going to be. The four of us.

"She sure is," Alf said, cupping her whole head in his palm. "Our little Dinky Dot."

Mam had given him a smile that looked tired and after a bit they laid her in the crib in the corner and I went out to play with Billy.

She'd not stayed that small for long, but as soon as she could walk she'd put her hand in mine and held on. I dragged her round the market, swung on the swings, played tag in the street. There was no more bombing or firing at Hitler as our games had moved on by then.

"Take your sister with you," Mam would say without fail if I put my shoes on. And there she'd be. Baby teeth and hot hands, trotting to keep up with me. Dinky Dot.

The hand in mine pulled me forward again and I looked to see if it was her. But it wasn't. It was the other one. Daisy. I blinked and was about to step further into the stream when Phyllis appeared on the bank and I knew from her face I was in the doghouse.

Nina

Nina was very rarely cold, probably because she was very rarely still. The rest of them were all bundled up in scarves and gloves and overcoats, and Freddie and Daisy wore wellington boots too and their cheeks were as pink as cherries under their woolly hats. Nina just wore her hoodie and her jeans and Dr. Martens. All in black, she could hardly be seen, which was just the way she liked it as they made their way around the dark park and towards the fire.

There was a crowd from college there. She'd seen them. Not with their families, like her. They were out with their mates or dates, the boys all in padded jackets and the girls wearing lip gloss. They pushed and jostled each other, some linked arms, the tallest boy threw an awkward arm round one of the girls. There was a bottle being passed around, although none of them were eighteen. They giggled and slipped and shrieked and loved the attention they got, the looks from the crowd. They were the pretty ones, the popular ones. The crowd she was not part of. She kept her head down as they passed.

The rev of an engine in the car park caught Nina's attention. A black motorbike was parked there, the rider sitting astride it with his back to her, revving it up to the nods and grunts of the surrounding group of boys. She saw Pops turn his head to the sound too and then he peeled away from Nan, who was chatting to Mum and didn't immediately notice. He edged over to the bike, right into the circle of boys, and joined in with the nodding and listening, as if he belonged there. Nina glanced anxiously at Nan, who was still moving obliviously forwards, and then back at Pops, who was gaining the attention of the group too. What should she do? The boys flicked glances at him and then nudged each other, smirks on their faces.

"Whatcha want, Grandad?" one of the boys said, and the others burst into laughter and doubled over as though it was hilarious. Without thinking Nina took the few steps towards Pops, put a hand on his elbow, almost – but not quite – in the ring herself. Pops had his head cocked on one side and then raised one gnarly old bent finger in the air. The rider revved the engine one more time and then everyone stared at Pops as the noise died. The rider took his helmet off and turned off the bike. Nina recognised him from the college canteen and felt a sinking feeling in her stomach. Could this get any worse?

She pulled gently at Pops' elbow, but he cleared his throat and said, "You want to check your bottom end."

Someone snorted and another laughed.

Nina wished she was anywhere else but there.

"Sorry, what?" the rider said.

"Something wrong with your arse apparently!" the gobby one said, and got a punch on the arm for being so funny.

Pops ignored him and squinted at the rider.

"I mean it," he said. "That knocking sound's not right."

"Who are you – the motorbike whisperer?" someone else said and everyone fell about.

"Don't leave it too long," Pops said with a shrug. "It can cause real problems."

"Pops," said Nina quietly, tugging his sleeve. The last thing she wanted was to draw the attention onto herself. He looked slightly surprised to see her there, but, to her relief, let her move him away a step, before turning again to the rider.

"If you don't know how to do it yourself, you could ask the BBC." He pointed his finger to make his point. Nina took the opportunity to lead him further away.

"Oh, of cooooooooouuuurse, mate," the mouthy one commented, behind them. "He could just ring up the BBC and ask the man on the television how to mend his noisy bottom!"

When Nina looked over her shoulder, the boys sounded and looked as stupid as a pack of hyenas. Suddenly she fizzed so much inside it spilled onto the outside. She spun on her heel and marched back towards the rider himself. Her feet crunched on the gravel and she saw his eyebrows go up in surprise.

"He means the Bromley Bike Club. The BBC. He set it up nearly fifty years ago and he knows everything there is to know about motorbikes. So, if he says your bottom end needs attention, it probably does. Like your attitude." Oh God, how had that happened? Nina realised she sounded like her mum. But she'd had to say something. It wasn't right for them to talk to him like that. She felt everyone's eyes on her.

There was a split second of silence.

Then the rider nodded at her, one quick dip of his head, and said, with a definite ring of approval, "Feisty."

And Nina blew all her air out in a huff as the others looked from one to another as if not sure what their response should be.

She strode away, grabbed Pops by the elbow and walked him slightly too fast towards the darkness of the park again.

"He needs to get that sorted," Pops said again to her, or himself, as he stumbled along beside her, and then, "Slow down a bit, TillyMint."

She exhaled as they reached the safety of the family gang again and realised only then her shoulders were back and she was standing tall. She'd never stood up for anyone before, and she'd definitely never been thought of as feisty.

Nina risked a glance back over her shoulder and to her surprise the motorbike boy was still sitting on his bike, watching her as he pulled a vape from a pocket of his leather jacket. He took a long drag and blew vapour out without taking his eyes off her. The smoky haze seemed to plume out of his mouth for ages. She felt pinned like a rabbit in a gun sight and so she turned away, although she sensed his eyes on her back. Oh my God, she'd seen that expression on the television before, just never in real life – not at her. He hadn't just looked at her, he'd looked *into* her. Almost as if he liked her. It meant all she could see in her mind was his eyes, not the little straggly beard she'd noticed when they were up close, nor the shape of his nose. Just his eyes as they held her. She wanted to run around, bounce, jump. She flapped her free hand fiercely by her side and led Pops on. A moment or two later she heard the motorbike start up again and ride away.

"There you are!" called Mum, and the moment was gone. "Take your hood down, Nina. You look like a gangster." The night air nipped down the back of her neck as her mum pushed the fabric off her head.

"Get off," Nina said, yanking it back up and hoping motorbike boy had looked away. "You've all got hats on. What's the difference?"

"There's a world of difference," her mum said. "And I DID leave a hat out for you, love."

Nina had seen it, laid out on the kitchen table. A pink woolly bobble hat. As though she were the same age as Freddie and Daise. There was absolutely no way she'd be seen dead in it. She turned her back on her mum and heard her sigh as she looked towards Nan and Pops before angling her head towards Jess and the kids.

"Are your feet warm now, Daisy?" Jess was asking. Daisy jumped up and down, full of hot chocolate and sugar – which Nina had definitely NOT been offered, but looking at Daisy she wanted to jump up and down too. She took Daisy's hands in hers and they jumped together. Daisy was squealing, breathless as they bounced round in a circle. Then Nina remembered the college group and checked they weren't looking. Two were standing looking at each other as if they were about to kiss. The others were sharing headphones and listening to music. She let go of Daisy's hands.

"You're so good with the kids," Jess said, nudging her gently. "Did you hear what Pops did earlier? Honestly, fancy taking Daisy in the river. I can't be doing with her getting a cold now, they won't let her in to nursery and then what will I do? Nan says he's just not making good decisions. It's the dementia."

Nina knew that feeling. Every decision she had to make felt like it was the biggest thing ever. Most decisions had too many options. The more options, the more nervous she got. The more nervous she got, the harder it was to make a choice. It wasn't just the big decisions like college or course, it was the smaller ones, like which sandwich to have or what programme to watch. Never films, they lasted too long and she couldn't keep her mind on them. She even found it hard to choose clothes to wear every day, so a uniform of jeans, hoodie and Doc Martens took the stress out of it. Mum used to try to buy her coloured tops and jackets but now she just did a dark wash twice a week and "was done with it". It felt like even Nina's fashion sense was a disappointment.

A family walked past, the kids holding sparklers out in front of them. They sparkled and glittered and Nina's insides lit up with them. Her hands fluttered again by her sides.

Daisy's eyes were as big as mirrors, and she spun on the spot to pull at Jess's arm.

"Mummy!" she said. "Mummy!"

Freddie was there out of nowhere, joining his sister.

"Mummy, can we have sparklers?"

Both of them together. "PLEASE!"

Nina wanted one too. She wanted to write her name on the air, smell the burning, spin in a circle and watch the trail above her head.

Jess looked across the crowd, peering towards the stall the other side of the fire.

"I can't see where they got them from, can you, Neen?"

Nina bounced foot to foot, side to side, suddenly very busy inside. But somehow feeling too as if she could do anything. After all, she'd just stood up to a bunch of boys being idiots to Pops.

"I could take them," she said. "I can find the stall."

Jess frowned, just slightly between her two perfect eyebrows.

"You just said I'm really good with the kids." Nina shoved her hands in her pockets to stop them moving. She had to make the outside match what she felt inside. She needed to look like she could achieve this. She could be "normal".

"I know," Jess said, "but the sparklers can give a really nasty burn – and we don't know how far away they are…"

"I'd be careful, Jess." Nina's hand broke free again, clenched and banging against her leg.

Jess looked away. Her eyes darted about and then alighted on something that made her smile. "But here's Andy now, look, he can go. Then you can stay and keep me company."

Nina felt the blood rush into her face as she looked at her beautiful, calm, non-weird older sister, who squeezed her arm.

At the same time, Nina heard an unmistakeable sound. A "cheep, cheep" from the cool crowd, who had now appeared by the fire. One glance told her they'd spotted her. A boy ran around with his arms out like a bird and a couple of the others whistled and tweeted in her direction.

She pulled her hood strings so tight that all that was left to see were her eyes. She sighed. Normal? Who was she kidding.

The Far Away

1949

Dot took to her feet for the first time holding my hand in the back room while Mam worked behind the counter in the shop. Her little sticky fingers clung tightly to mine as she padded a few steps before dropping to her knees and gurgling wet and happy in my direction.

After that, she'd walk for hours pointing chubby fingers and dimpled knuckles where she wanted to go next. The corner. The door. The window. Then I'd pull her up onto the chair with me so we could press our noses to the glass and watch Main Street. Sometimes she'd fall asleep there and suck her thumb till Mam came and put her in the pram to go home. At night she was my "own personal bed warmer" according to Mam. Which was fine till her nappy was heavy and wet and smelled like vinegar. Thankfully, she'd grown out of that now. It was just the pillow got wet with her thumb-sucking. I liked to wake in the night to the constant sound of her soothing herself; it put me back to sleep too.

We'd moved back to Divine Street when Alf and Mam got married. I loved being back next door but one to Billy Sankey. We'd play out in the street, even if we did have Dot and his little brother Sammy trailing along beside us.

Everyone was used to seeing Liberty parked outside of ours at night. And they all knew to leave it alone. Even George Malone since I punched him in the nose. I still grinned at the thought of his surprised face. His eyebrows almost hit his hairline as he felt my fist in his face. He gave me a wide berth these days. Alf had banged me on the back when I told him. "That's my boy," he said even though I knew I wasn't. But it was nice of him to say it all the same.

One Sunday in summer, the air was so heavy and hot that Dinky was outside in her pants and Sammy wore his birthday suit. Mammy pinched her mouth together when she saw he didn't even have his drawers on, but didn't say anything at all. She sat on the doorstep with Alf, the same as all the other grown-ups. A day off. A public holiday they called it. A scorcher. Alf drank beer with the men. Mammy sipped on a sherry. Her cheeks were flushed and it wasn't just the heat.

Billy and I played British Bulldog and Tag and skimmed stones across the cobbles like we had done all summer. Dinky and Sammy tried to skim but their stones bounced and died. Dot really didn't care. She was grinning at the noise each one made as it hit the floor. She'd grin at me as if she'd done well and I could only nod back in encouragement to make her happy.

It was different that day, playing out while the adults were there. We hung round the edges of them, watching them get louder and laugh harder as the day went on. Someone put his or her wireless in the window and then there was music too.

It was almost teatime when Alf jumped up and slapped his thigh in excitement.

"For one night only…" he said, his voice booming down the street. Everyone turned his way.

"The circus is coming to town!"

He raised both hands in the air theatrically and then bowed. Mam rolled her eyes and giggled.

Alf disappeared in the doorway, practically climbing over Mam as she sat there, and reappeared seconds later jangling Liberty's keys. I threw my stone to the gutter, more interested in him and the bike.

"Alf..." Mam said but he just laughed and said, to everyone now watching:

"The most daring family show!"

I bit my lip. Not sure what he was talking about, "family show", but also not sure if he meant me as well. I knew there was a difference between Dot and me. She called him Dad. I called him Alf.

He strode over to Liberty and someone started a slow clap. Alf threw his thigh over the saddle, kicked the stand with the heel of his boot and walked the bike away from the kerb.

"Josie," he called to Mam. She waved him away with one hand, laughed with Mrs Sankey.

"A family show's never complete without the mam!" Alf said and beckoned her with one finger. It was like a worm hooking at her and pulling her in.

She stood and smoothed her skirt down as she moved towards him, as though hypnotised. She couldn't stay away.

"Never seen before this side of the Mersey!" Alf called and people stood in the doorways now to see what he was up to. I leaned against the wall, waiting to see too.

"Grab Dottie!" he said and Mammy scooped her up in her pants and they both made their way towards him. Something hurt in my chest. I pushed myself further into the shadow of the terrace, bricks hard against my spine.

"Climb on," he said to Mam and shuffled back on Liberty, making room for her at the front of the saddle. She squeezed in between his body and the handlebars, with Dot sitting right at the front of them all. Alf reached round Mam and tickled Dot in the ribs and she squealed and put her hands on the grips. I knew that tickle almost hurt, he'd done it to me before. My stomach twisted and I felt my ears go red. I hoped nobody was looking at me.

"Liverpool's one and only… Daredevil family!" Alf announced. Mr Sankey did three cheers and raised his tankard in the air and still nobody mentioned me.

Alf pushed the bike a little bit further up the street, moving towards the middle of the cobbles. Billy Sankey ran to remove Sammy Sankey, who was walking starkers up the street in pursuit. He picked him up to carry him away and everyone laughed at Sammy's white bum.

"Put it away!" someone called.

Alf turned the key. Liberty roared. Everyone cheered. My eyes got hot and I blinked quickly.

Suddenly Alf killed the engine. He looked round behind him and then shook his head. Turning my way, he pointed straight at me.

"What you doing over there, Ernie?" He laughed and thumbed over his shoulder. "You're meant to be on the back!"

Everyone laughed and I made a funny noise. A hiccup or a laugh. Or a sob of relief. I'm not sure. But I made it to the bike in a couple of steps. He hoisted me over the saddle at the back and then grinned at me.

"Stand up then, son," he said, quietly, to me.

"What?" said Mam at the front, cricking her neck to hear.

"Nothing love," Alf said to her and then nodded to me to climb up. He winked as I bit my lip, and that was all it took. "Hold on here," he said, putting my hands on his shoulders.

"I haven't got a helmet on," I said.

"Never mind that, just this once," he said. "Like I said, it's for One Night Only!" He said the last words loudly, so that the whole terrace could hear, and I put my shaky feet on the saddle, one either side of his hips. My legs shook as I stood up behind him, holding onto his shoulders, feeling like my head was far too high off the ground and my feet were not balanced right. I saw Billy Sankey's eyes go wide.

Alf started the engine again. Libby backfired and the whole street ducked and screamed. Mrs Sankey laughed at the shock on her husband's face. "Don't worry love, it's not a bomb!" she told him and he clapped himself on the chest like he was having a heart attack.

Then we were off.

Liberty bumped over the cobbles slowly but surely. Alf stuck his legs out the sides of the bike like a clown. His massive feet turned upwards towards the sky between the rows of houses. Mam laughed up front and said, "not too fast," and Alf said to "stop worrying," while Dinky squealed and banged her hands on the handlebars.

And I stood up as straight as I could, terrified and as excited as I'd ever been. The feel of the bike beneath me made my breath catch but Alf's shoulders felt steady and safe under my hands. The sun was shining on my face and the terrace clapped and cheered as we rode past. I saw Billy's face, mouth as wide as his eyes now.

I gasped as we hit a cobble and jolted just enough to make the crowd gasp and then clap. We did one way up to Welbeck Street and then back down again and I wished it would never end. It was the happiest I'd ever felt in my life.

Christmas 1950 was my tenth Christmas and suddenly I stood taller than Alf's waist. Everyone in the terrace asked me if I'd been standing with my feet in a bucket of manure, I was growing so quickly. I studied my face in the square of mirror in the lavatory to see if I still looked the same as my arms and legs got longer and I hardly knew what they were doing half the time. But much to my disappointment, my ears continued to stick out of my head, not growing upwards like the rest of me. I pressed them in with my hands until they went red in the hope that they might stick.

Alf had started a fruit and veg stall at the market. He spent all the savings he had on a barrow, his first load and buying a cheap pitch at the edge of the market.

Then, little by little, as people moved on or died, he edged himself into a better position until soon he was on Main Street itself, right by the pub and the baker. Handy for the women to buy their veggies at the same time as their bread, he used to say with a wink at me, or for the men to pick a little something up on the way home to keep the women happy. A punnet of strawberries or a sweet red apple to make someone smile. His early-morning start on the market meant he was up before the birds each day. He headed to the fruit market in the coldest, darkest hours to select the best stock for his stall. By the time I went to school, his working day was half done.

The Everyday and Far Away

I could hear him as I walked to school in the mornings, calling out to passers-by.

"Penny a pound!" he'd say. Or, "Morning Mrs Johnson, what can I tempt you with today?" Alf always knew everyone's name and their favourite items and of course he'd add an extra cherry for the little one hanging off her mother's skirts. And he'd bring anything home with him that couldn't be sold the next day, and Mam would cut it up for us to try. I still didn't eat bananas though.

There was frost on the back steps on Christmas morning and the air plumed like I was smoking a cigarette as I ran to the toilet. I showed Dot, posing with my fingers in the air as if they held a fag. She laughed and copied me, walking with a wiggle down the path, like the women at the docks. She blew out imaginary smoke as she went, leaving tiny little footprints in the white sparkling ground.

Dot was still tiny. When we got back in the house, Alf swung her up to sit on his shoulder and she'd put her hands up to touch the ceiling. She perched there like a little bird, and sometimes that would make me wish I were still little too.

We each had a satsuma in our stocking and we peeled them in front of the fire. The peel hissed as we threw it onto the coals and it curled up in a tight black ball. But it scented the room with the sweetest fragrance.

"That's the smell of Christmas," said Mam as she leaned against Alf on the sofa. He smiled with pleasure and had a doze while Dot and I sucked the flesh of each individual segment of fruit until we were left with a little empty sack. I flicked mine at her and she giggled when it stuck on her hand. She tried to flick hers back at me but her little-girl fingers didn't have the same kick in them that mine did.

The next day I woke up to a cold, wet bed. I grimaced and moved to push Dot with my feet to get her up and out of the bed, but my feet landed on her shins under the blanket and she was as hot as the coal had been the night before. I crawled down the bed to her head end and her cheeks were scarlet, her eyelashes fluttering on them like black spiders.

Mam took charge. I was to sleep on the sofa for a few nights to give Dottie the bed. Mam sponged her down with a rag and cold water, and she opened the window even though it made me shiver. I could see when she spoke to Dot as her breath showed white in the air. I was sent in and out with errands. I had to collect some chicken bones from the butcher's so that Mam could make a broth. Take the soiled rags out of the room. Take some clean water in for Dot to drink. I hesitated by her bed, but Mam shooed me away. Dottie didn't know I was there anyway, she slept and moaned around the thumb in her mouth.

"It's everywhere," I heard Alf say to Mam that night as he prepared to get into bed, hanging his waistcoat over the back of the armchair, slipping out of his braces.

Mam clenched her hands in front of her, the lamp throwing shadows under her face until I thought she looked like an old, old woman. I looked away, frightened to see her like that.

"It's all the market's talking about," he said. "Worst flu in years." Mammy kept looking towards Dottie's door. "People dropping like flies."

Mam wrung her hands like she still had a rag between them.

"You don't think…" she said, quietly but Alf pulled her into a hug and whatever she said was muffled into his chest.

"She'll be fine," he said, clearly, into the top of her head. I saw her hands hold onto him, and when she let go his shirt was all crumpled into creases.

The next day, Dottie died. Very quietly, without ever once having come out of her bedroom alive since Christmas. Mam and Alf got very busy just before it happened, and the doctor came in to see her, but there was nothing to be done. I was kept out of the room, but the walls were thin and Mammy made a noise that made the hair on my neck stand up and I didn't know whether to stay where I was or go in to see her. In the end, I waited and Mam came out to say I could say my goodbyes. I didn't really know what she meant till she nudged me towards the bedroom door and my belly sank as she led me towards the bed.

Dottie looked like she'd gone to sleep and forgotten to come back. The bit that made her Dottie, even when she was sleeping, was gone. I stared at her hand and thought it would never try to flick a piece of satsuma at me again. Or skim a stone. Or hold my fingers on the way home from school. I put my hand out to touch hers but then stopped. I didn't want to feel it cold.

Alf carried her to the undertakers himself, wrapped in a blanket. The whole street stood on their doorsteps as he went past. Mrs Sankey cried. I heard her call out to Alf but he didn't speak in return.

Mam took to her bed and I heard her weeping through the wall. Alf, for a very loud man, cried very quietly. When he came back he sank into his chair by the fire, the tears streaming off his big red nose and dripping to his chest.

And after the crying stopped, the house was the quietest I'd ever known.

Until Mam started coughing.

*

Mam's cough got worse. It started off harsh-sounding. Like it was too big and nasty to have come out of her body. She was only little, my mam. But her cough was huge and it hacked through the wall as I lay in bed. Alf sat beside her and then slept in the armchair when he couldn't keep his eyes open any more. He opened the stall the first day, leaving me on duty with Mam. I kept the window open like he told me, sponged her face with a cold cloth every now and then, and lifted her head to sip at the water when she called for it. Her eyes were dark as a blackbird's, and they never seemed to settle on me for long. It was like she was looking for something. Or someone. But sometimes, she'd put a hand out to me, like I could help her. She'd say Dottie's name like she'd just remembered. And then she'd cry until she coughed again. I wiped her brow but never knew what to say. Even if I had the words, I'd not be able to say them over the Dottie-sized lump in my throat.

I was glad when Alf got home. He went straight to her room and then told me I'd done a good job. Although the words were nice to hear, his voice was sad.

Over the next few days, Mam's cough got weaker. It sounded like her body couldn't be bothered to do it any more. Alf brought the doctor in the next afternoon. They talked on the landing outside her door and when the doctor let himself out I saw Alf lay his head against the closed door and shut his eyes. I hurt all over when he did that.

The next day when I came home from school, Alf was at the kitchen table with his head in his hands.

I ran towards Mam's bedroom but he put a giant hand out to stop me.

"She's gone, lad," he said.

I didn't believe him. For where was she going to go, what with having the flu? It wasn't like she could go far. I pushed past him and opened the bedroom door and the bed was empty. All the sheets rolled back and stripped. As if she'd never been there at all.

The Everyday

"All right, Dad?" Sue said, sitting in the armchair next to mine. She was all smiles and bosom, not that I was meant to say things like that. She rolled her eyes if I dared.

"What's new then?" she said. I hate it when she asks bloody silly questions like that. I whistled a few notes and she smiled.

"Always were a good whistler, Dad, weren't you?"

I whistled a few more to see if she'd stop asking questions.

She sat back in the chair and I breathed a sigh of relief, focused on the telly, leaving Phyllis and her a little girl-time.

There were some children on the TV, a whole group of them running up a hill somewhere, singing. As if that would bloody happen. I'd not have been running about singing when I was a boy. Once I grew out of pretending to bomb the Jerries, I liked throwing stones at the empty dock buildings. We used to go down there on the weekends, a whole gang of us. Me and Billy Sankey and anyone else that wanted to come along. We knew we'd be battered if anyone realised what we were up to.

"I had the best score for smashing windows on the whole street by the time I was eleven," I said. Sue and Phyllis stopped talking and turned to me.

"What's that, love?" Phyllis said.

I grinned and she patted my hand on the armrest of my chair.

"The best score," I said again.

"At what, Dad?" Sue asked.

"What?" I said back.

Sue sighed. "I bet you did, Dad, you were always good at it."

I didn't know what she was saying I was good at so I whistled a little more and she smiled back.

The kids on the television were now climbing trees, which was more like it. But they were still bloody singing. Some of them tall strong boys too. What on earth would their dad be thinking of them, running around the countryside singing and dancing. Surely they should be signed up for national service soon? The size of them.

"I did the service you know," I said but neither of them heard me. Their heads close together, Phyllis's hair white as snow. When did that happen? Mind you, I thought I could see a bit of grey at Sue's temple too. Who'd have thought that I could be old enough to have a daughter with hair that colour.

"Stephen should have done the service too," I said and then they both turned to me again. Quicker this time.

"They'd stopped it by then though, hadn't they, love?" Phyllis said.

"What'd they do that for? Best thing for a boy," I said, wagging my finger at the television as the boys ran around in shorts made of some flowery material. "That lot'd do well to go too."

Sue smiled at me, but it wasn't a big grin, and she wiped her eye as she turned back to her mam. I didn't know she suffered from hay fever.

Now there was a Nazi flag on the screen and I watched as an old car drove along, a man wearing a uniform got out and did the *Sieg Heil*.

"Pah," I snorted.

"Turn it over if you don't want to watch it, love," said Phyllis.

I ignored her, hoping she'd do it but she was talking again. I listened in for a bit to see what had them gossiping.

"He keeps getting up at four a.m.," she said and Sue patted her arm.

"Must be ingrained, Mum, he did it for so many years on the market or the shop. You can't blame him for that."

Who keeps getting up at 4a.m.? Was she talking about Alf? He used to be up before the dawn chorus. I cleared my throat and did the whistle of a blackbird.

"Blackbird," Sue said immediately. She was a good girl, my Sue.

I turned back to the television but kept half an ear on them to see if she whistled one back to me.

"But he gets up and gets dressed and then I have to persuade him to come back to bed. Then he does it again an hour later. And again. By the time my alarm actually goes off, we're both exhausted," Phyllis said.

I whistled again.

"Mistle thrush," Sue said and I stuck two thumbs up at her.

The programme on the telly was getting a bit soppy. There was a woman playing a guitar and singing as all the children sat round her. She had nice eyes but her haircut was shocking. I looked over at Sue's hair again, at the bit of white on the side, and opened my mouth. Then I shut it again. I kept saying the wrong thing apparently and it was better if I whistled at her. She smiled when I did that.

"I honestly don't know what to do with her," Sue was moaning now to Phyllis. "I had another call from the college yesterday."

"What now?" Phyllis said.

"Same old thing. Not finishing work. Not handing it in. Not listening. She's literally hanging on by her fingernails." Sue blew out all the air in her body in one long blow. "The teachers all agree she's bright enough. But she's constantly distracted. And not necessarily by something else going on around her. Nina can literally distract herself in an empty room by what's going on inside her head."

"Have you talked to her about it?" Phyllis asked.

"She never seems to want to. She said she's fed up it seems to be so easy for some people to learn things. How they hear something once and they know it. But she says that she can't get her brain to listen properly. It must be so frustrating."

"I'm sure fidgety people in our school were just tied to their chair," said Phyllis, but Sue didn't seem to think that was very helpful.

"It's not just fidgeting, Mum…" Sue sighed.

"I know, love," Phyllis said. "She can't help it. It's the ABC."

"ADHD, Mum. ADHD. Attention Deficit Hyperactivity Disorder. Anyway, I'm not tying Nina down anywhere. I just wish it wasn't so hard for her. I think it might be time to talk about medication. We always said it was a last resort but maybe we're getting to that stage."

"Give the doctors a ring. They might be able to help. Maybe ask them at the same time if they can give me something to keep your dad in the bed till a more decent time."

I stretched my feet out in front of me and wiggled my toes. Dottie used to do that in the bed to see if the bed was warm or not, and then tuck them back up underneath her bottom with a "brrr".

The Everyday and Far Away

The fire in the lounge was making me sleepy. I liked having a bit of a sleep in the afternoons in the chair but lately Phyllis had been waking me up all the time. Saying I'd sleep better later when I went to bed. Bloody annoying. Every time I nodded off, she nudged me with her elbow.

"Do you want to stay for some tea, Sue?" Phyllis said and my stomach rumbled. It seemed a long time since lunch. I couldn't even remember what she'd made me.

"No, I need to get back. I'm minding Daisy and Fred tomorrow for Jess. So I've got to get everything ready for school in the morning."

"You're a good girl, Susie," Phyllis said, patting her hand on the arm of the chair as she stood. Sue looked pleased as she heaved herself upwards too.

"You going on the school bus?" I asked her. I'd seen her on the back seat once as it drove past, she was smoking. Never told her mum, who'd have been furious.

Sue laughed. "Not any more, Dad," she said, pulling on her coat. "Anyway. Better go." She kissed me on the head as she went past and Phyllis stood to walk her to the front door.

"Bye Dad," she said. "Love you."

"Bye," I said.

Sue paused for a moment like she was waiting for something and then went out.

I glared at the television. A concert hall. Lots of people singing a song I didn't know. What were they doing that for? It wasn't our national anthem or anything. I knew "God Save the Queen", every word of it, and this wasn't it.

I snorted. "Bloody rubbish."

"If you don't like it," Phyllis said, as she came back in, "change it."

She handed me a black plastic thing, with coloured buttons on it, squiggles and signs. I put it on the arm of the chair and waited for her to turn the telly over for me. "Want to watch *Wanted Down Under?*" Phyllis asked.

"What's that?" I said. There was a blackbird on the feeding table outside the window. Its beak bright yellow.

"*Wanted Down Under?*" she said again, pointing to something in the *Radio Times*. "Starts in two minutes."

She settled herself in the armchair next to mine, always on my right so I could reach over and hold her hand. She liked that. I liked it too. It took her a moment to fiddle with some buttons but then the TV changed channels.

"It's all about people going to Australia, remember? Or sometimes New Zealand. You know?"

The music started on the TV and Phyllis sighed.

I turned back to the screen. To the smiling host and a sunny day. I was going to New Zealand once. Or Australia. One or the other, I can't remember which. It was a long time ago.

Nina

Her mother was in the kitchen when Nina got home from college. The eighties radio station was on and Sue was singing along and throwing her hips about as she smoothed mashed potato onto the top of a cottage pie. Or shepherd's pie. Whichever it was, the kitchen smelled good and Nina chucked her rucksack behind the door and pulled up a chair at the small, wooden kitchen table instead of running straight outside to the trampoline. She wanted to be near her mum and she hoped she could stay still long enough that her mum might give her a cuddle. It had been one of those days. In fact, they all felt like one of those days at the moment.

Mum raised her hands above her head, waving her spatula, old-person dancing to the electro beats.

"First band I ever saw," she said as the song ended. "Thompson Twins. Hammersmith Apollo. 1984." Her eyes went all faraway for a second and then she licked the spatula, tossed it in the sink and turned the radio down a notch. "You all right, love?"

Nina weighed up the question in her head. It wasn't as straightforward as it sounded. She bit her lip. Everything was in a muddle. She opened her mouth but nothing came out.

"College okay?" Sue prompted, pushing the pie into the oven, then turning to look at her daughter properly.

Nina felt her eyes get hot and the flush of heat in her cheeks and then to her horror she was crying. Great noisy gulps and runny nose, the lot. Her mum was across the kitchen in a second, swallowing her up in a big, hot hug. "Oh, love," she murmured into Nina's hair until the storm had passed. Eventually, Nina sat back and Sue pulled out the chair next to her, knees touching. She didn't even try to stop Nina's knee from doing its own little jig.

"Is it college?"

Nina nodded with a sniff. Of course it was.

"Well, whatever's happened, we can work it out."

Although she was saying the right words, Nina could see the worry behind the smile and the sight just made her feel worse. Why couldn't she just be normal? Then nobody would have to worry so much. She wiped her nose on the back of her hand and her mum passed her a tissue from the box.

"So, what's going on, Neen? I mean, *really* going on?"

"I'm just so behind, Mum." Nina balled the soggy tissue in her hand. "In everything."

Her mum opened her mouth, but Nina carried on.

"And I don't like my courses…"

Sue tilted her head to one side, sensing there was more.

"And I haven't got any friends…"

Sue pressed her lips together as though she might cry herself and Nina said the last thing.

"And I'm just too… *weird*." Her voice broke on the word and her mum leaned across, and this time it was a proper bear hug.

"Right, Nina. That's a lot all at once. For anyone. So, let's do one thing at a time."

Nina's breath hitched with every inhale as she listened.

"First of all, and most importantly, you are *not* weird."

Nina sighed.

"You're *not*," Sue reiterated, pressing Nina's hand to emphasise it. "You are a very normal seventeen-year-old girl, with hormones and worries and hopes."

"And ADHD…"

"And ADHD," agreed Sue with a shrug. "But I'm sure there are other people there with ADHD. How are they getting on?"

Nina blew out between her lips in frustration. "I don't know, Mum, we don't have an ADHD club, you know."

Her mum sat back at the dig, but then tried again.

"I just mean that everyone has their own things to work with, to overcome," she said, quietly. "And just because you have ADHD it doesn't mean you're weird. You're a kind, funny girl who tries really hard. Who just also happens to have ADHD."

Nina wished she could believe her.

"You could always try the medication if you thought—"

Nina banged her hand on her own thigh. "So, one minute I'm normal and the next you're suggesting I change myself with some medicine."

"I don't want to change you for the world, love," Sue said. "I love you very much. It's completely your choice."

"Then I want to be me," Nina said, even though she wasn't at all sure who that was just yet. Sue squeezed her hand again. "No pills."

They eyed each other for a moment and then Mum nodded at her decision.

"So, the courses? If you don't like yours, is there another course you'd rather do? Should we look into changing?"

This was new. Nina raised her eyebrows, surprised. She had expected her mother to give the normal spiel about how they'd chosen them as the best of a bad bunch, and she should stick things out, and now Nina found she didn't know what to say.

"That's the problem," she said. "I might not like the ones I'm doing, but I don't like any of the others either."

Sue nodded and thought for a moment.

"Some people just aren't at their best at school," she said eventually. She reached her hand out and tried to tuck Nina's hair behind her ear, where it never normally went.

"College," Nina corrected, shaking her hair free again without meaning to. Mum ignored the interruption.

"Like Jeremy Clarkson," she said with a knowing look. "He failed his exams you know, and look at him now."

Nina blinked, trying to see how a middle-aged guy who wore checked shirts and drove cars was in any way like her.

"Sometimes, you just have to get through this bit and then you find your way afterwards..." Sue clarified.

"What? Find my passion?" Nina said, without intending her sarcastic tone, but still she got a definitive nod back.

"So, if it's a case of getting through this phase..." Sue said. "How can I help you get through easier?"

Nina shook her head.

"For example, you said you're behind? Can I help with that? Maybe some planning or better time organisation? There's this thing on Facebook where you can think of your time in fifteen-minute blocks and do something constructive with each of them. We could make up a planner and work out when you're doing what."

Before Sue had finished speaking Nina was already trying to work out how many fifteen-minute blocks there were in a day and thinking she could easily waste fifteen minutes looking for the pen she'd lose when she was trying to fill in the planner in the first place. She sighed, bringing herself back to the present. Her mum was still looking at her, hopeful, waiting.

She wanted to say thanks for the thought, or something kind, but instead heard herself push her mother away. "It's not up to you, though. I should be doing this on my own."

"I know, but everyone needs a hand sometimes."

Nina's eyes filled up again. Why was she being so horrible?

"Is there anyone at college you could talk to? Would that be better?"

Nina sniffed. Nodded. "They do this thing where they pair you up and you can talk to a Year 13. So I've put my name down and asked for a mentor to help me."

Her mum reacted like Nina had found a cure for world peace.

"There you go," she said, nudging Nina's shoulder. "That will help and that's you doing it all on your own. Let's see what she says about it. Then, you let me know if you need me to help as well. I'm always here."

Nina took a deep breath and acknowledged to herself that what her mum said was true.

She *had* enquired about it on her own. Maybe it *would* help.

"And don't worry about not making friends immediately. It's always better if it takes time, otherwise you might pair up with someone you liked at first and then realise she's not your type and then you're stuck with them for good!" Sue laughed as though Nina had the pick of friends at college and she could take her time to choose. "You'll find the right one!"

Nina flashed back to her lunchtime sitting on her own in the canteen, hearing the occasional "cheep" or "tweet-tweet" from other students. The only slightly disconcerting thing had been today when the motorbike boy from the fireworks came in with his mates. He carried his white motorbike helmet in his hand, and Nina could see he'd written **SPLAT HAT** on the top of it in black sharpie. She imagined the motorbike parked in the college car park outside.

He'd bought a portion of chips at the serving hatch and she saw the dinner lady shake her head and roll her eyes as he walked away although she couldn't hear what he'd said. He'd thrown a good few of the chips at his mates as they lounged in the corner, some sitting on the backs of chairs rather than the seats, and they'd shared the rest before he lobbed the empty box at a nearby bin, where it hit the rim and fell to the floor. A passing teacher pointed at him and then the litter and he dragged himself to his feet as his friends laughed.

But as he straightened up from picking up the rubbish he had spotted Nina watching from her place by the window. A flash of recognition passed over his face and a hint of surprise, Nina thought, that she was there. His cheeks flushed as he tried to puff up his chest and suddenly Nina felt sorry for his embarrassment. And without meaning to, she smiled.

His eyes widened, and then he dropped his forehead slightly and fixed her with that stare again, as he rolled the paper in his hands and luckily, this time, threw a perfect shot at the bin. The chip wrapper landed without touching the sides. His friends cheered and he winked at her before turning back to them.

Nina realised her mouth was open and quickly closed it. She grabbed her bag, her only thought to get out of the canteen and

The Everyday and Far Away

do laps of the campus. Anywhere she could move, walk, run. She wasn't sure – because she didn't dare look back – but she thought she could still feel his eyes on her as she pulled open the door to leave.

"There is one boy…" she said now to Sue, and then immediately wished she hadn't as she saw the glint of excitement in Sue's eyes.

"A boy? What's his name?"

Nina shook her head, not because she didn't want to say, but because she didn't know. But she didn't want her mum to know that.

"What's he like then?"

Nina shook her head again. She didn't know that either, apart from he was a crap shot and had a motorbike with a problem back end.

"All right, you don't have to tell me!" Mum said with a smile.

The phone rang and, as her mother went to answer it, Nina could imagine her having this conversation a hundred times with Jess, who had been popular at school before she settled down with Andy. The normality of it was nice.

Nina grinned at how good it actually felt to please her mum. Really make her happy. To see her smile like that. It felt like it had been ages since they'd been relaxed with each other. It gave her a rush inside and she wanted it to carry on, for Mum always to look at her like that. Not the worried lines, or the irritated frown. Just a delight. A smile.

"Oh, hello," Mum said cheerfully. "How did it go?" She frowned a little as she listened. Nina knew it was Nan as she and Sue always spoke at teatime every night.

Nina wondered whether her mum would want to ring her every day in the years to come, when they lived in different houses. She realised that she hoped it would be the case.

"Ah, that's good. So you both enjoyed it!" Sue looked at Nina and mouthed, "they've been to the cinema!" And then turned her attention back to the phone and said, "Yes, a good day here too! I've just been hearing that Nina's got her eye on a lad. Yes! I know!"

Nina felt the heat in her face but couldn't stop smiling as she stood and then headed for the trampoline.

The Far Away

1951

"Is he putting you in the orphanage then?" George Malone whispered as he went past on the way to school. My stomach went to water. He was the second person to say it that day. I had no fight left in me for George Malone that day so I just put my head down and carried on. He laughed and ran off.

It had been a whole month without Mam. Five weeks without Dot's feet pointing up towards me in the bed at night. All that extra space I had and I still stayed on my side. Not wanting to move over where she'd once been. It didn't seem fair to do that.

Alf made us things to eat in the evening, like bread and dripping or chops and potatoes depending on what he'd picked up on the way home. Sometimes Mrs Sankey helped out, bringing us a pie. His big face seemed to have fallen in on itself and he'd become very quiet. I caught him looking at me sometimes, like he was trying to answer a question in his head, and the look on his face made me drop my eyes. What was he seeing? What was he thinking?

He started going to the pub after tea. He'd pick up his overcoat and be half out the door before he remembered me there.

"See ya Ernie," he'd say. Or, "See you later, lad." He'd try to hold my eyes but his would slide off. It felt like I was holding my breath a lot of the time. While he was gone, Mrs Sankey would come and check on me and give me a hug. I'd always hold on, wanting the contact, but afterwards it would make me sad, because she didn't hug the same as Mam.

Alf slept in the chair more than he slept in his bed. I'd hear him snoring there when he came in from the pub. In the morning I'd hear his heavy feet staggering to the lav and back before he shut the front door, off to the stall. Then the day would start all over again. But there was a feeling in me that something was happening. Something was changing. I didn't know what, but I knew that nothing would ever be the same again.

Billy Sankey said it to me out loud when we were coming back from our paper rounds. We used to do our deliveries, him out towards the docks, me in towards the market, and then we'd meet on the corner and walk home together.

"Do you think he'll keep you then?" he said, blowing on his fingers to warm them up. They were purple poking out of his fingerless gloves.

I felt the words drop inside me. They'd been the ones in my own head for weeks.

"Seeing as he's not your dad and all?"

I shrugged although I felt like crying.

"Dunno," I said. "What do you think?"

Billy kicked a stone along the pavement and it ricocheted off the wall. Seemed like he didn't know what to say to that either.

I tried to make the tea that night. I spread some dripping thick and gloopy on a wedge of bread. I got a few rashers of bacon and fried them on the hob, dodging the fat as it spat at my hands. Alf raised a big bushy eyebrow when he saw it, and pulled out a chair. He demolished the plate in five minutes and wiped his mouth on the back of his hand. I wondered if it would be a good time to ask him if he had any plans for me. But he stood and put on his overcoat and I pressed my lips together tight. His eyes were a bit wet when he looked back at me.

"See you, Ernie," he said and took himself off to the pub.

The next night I told him a joke, even though I didn't really feel like laughing. Thought if I could make him happy, he'd be more likely to want me around.

"Where do you find a cow with no legs?" I said as he wiped a bit of bread and butter round the plate to sop up his gravy. My voice was a bit gruff as we weren't doing much talking in the house lately. He looked at me nonplussed so I cleared my throat and asked him again and then he stuffed the bread in his mouth and spoke around it.

"I don't know, where do you find a cow with no legs?"

"Right where you left it," I said and forced a grin.

He looked surprised for a minute and then a real laugh came out of him. A proper one. Not one of the ones when he looked at the ceiling and showed us all his tonsils. But a laugh all the same.

"Good one," he said, standing up. "See you later, lad."

I sighed. He still didn't want to stay home with me.

The next night, he didn't come back from the stall.

I waited until it was teatime and then set out to look for him. Barry Benny off the market told me to try the Fountain so I pressed my face to the window and there he was. At a table in the corner with a man I'd never seen before. There was money on the table in front of them and Alf was counting it out, coin by coin. Note by note. It looked like a lot. Something about the way he was counting it out, licking his fingers to separate the notes, checking the coins in each pile, made me nervous. I didn't go in.

If he'd sold me, I'd rather he told me when he got home. Then at least people wouldn't be looking at me.

He came home late and snored loudly that night. Like he'd had an extra pint. I curled on my side of the bed and wished Dot was there. The thought of her feet in the bed always made my eyes get hot, although eventually I'd fall asleep.

The next morning I found the leaflet on the floor by Alf's chair. It must have fallen out of his trouser pocket. I picked it up and smoothed it out. The picture caught my eye. A drawing of a boat. A child waving his hand in the air, a suitcase beside him on the deck.

I took it to the table and sat down.

The child had curly hair and chubby cheeks. His smile made dimples. The sun was out in the sky but he still wore his good coat. It was buttoned up.

A new life! the leaflet said on the front in bold lettering. I opened it up and there were more pictures. Children walking down a road swinging their bags. A map of a place I didn't know.

"Australia awaits!" it said.

My mouth went dry.

I read slowly, running my finger underneath each word, to be sure I was getting it right.

> *Families are waiting for children in Australia. A new life on a farm or community gives new opportunity to every child. Passage on board included. Children matched to the right home.*

The words swam in front of my eyes. Australia. Had Alf bought me a ticket? I remembered Mrs Finch in school spinning the atlas to show us Australia on the opposite side of the world.

She said it was night-time there when we had a day. That they had a winter when we were all out playing in the sun. That they had kangaroos and kookaburras and other things I'd never heard of. I wondered when he'd tell me.

I screwed the leaflet up as small as it would go and stuffed it in my trouser pocket. All day I felt it crinkle there as I moved in my chair at school. I didn't dare touch it again, or read it, in case I made something happen. I didn't tell Billy about it in case it came true.

Alf was packing a suitcase when I got home and I made my jaw as hard as it could be. I wouldn't cry. Not even if nobody else was looking.

"Sit down lad," he said, pulling out a chair for himself at the table.

"Things are different here now" – he cleared his throat – "what with your mam and Dottie gone."

I picked at the table with my nail. Pick, pick, pick.

"So I had to make some decisions about the future."

I got my fingertip under a splodge of stain on the top. Pick, pick, pick.

"We can't stay here, lad," he said, looking around him. I followed his look around the room. The hearth for the spitting games. The rug where Dottie and I played acrobats, me balancing her on my knees as she stood up as straight and tall as she ever got. The chair where Alf stretched his legs towards the fire. The table Mam wiped every night for crumbs.

Alf's eyes had big shadows underneath them and I saw just how tired he was. He probably hadn't had a proper sleep for weeks. He passed his great hands across his face, as though trying to rub everything away.

"I don't want to go," I said, not able to stop myself any more.

He looked at me through his fingers.

"You don't even know where, yet, lad—" he said.

"Australia!" I said, pulling the leaflet out of my pocket. I hurled it in a ball at him and it bounced off his chest. "They don't even have it cold at Christmas."

"Eh?" he said, opening the paper ball in front of him and squinting at it for a moment. His face shot upwards to look at me.

"Maybe Mrs Sankey will have me?" I said suddenly and his mouth dropped open a bit. I wondered if he hadn't thought of that. My chest tightened. I wouldn't mind sharing a bed with Billy. Not really. It would be better than going off on that boat on my own to live with the kangaroos.

"What are you talking about, Ernie?" Alf asked, putting the leaflet back down on the tabletop.

"That." I pointed. "You sending me off to Australia. I saw you with that man and the money in the Fountain and I know you've sold me" – he sat back in his chair like he'd been pushed – "but then I found this!" I pointed again. "You've bought me a ticket to a new life!" My eyes flashed hot and I blinked. It was the wrong thing to do as it made my tears overflow and run down my face. I swiped at them, angry with myself as much as him.

"That's just some rubbish," Alf said, "Some do-gooder down the pub gave it to me." He shook his head. "You're not going to Australia."

I gulped. Swallowed. Sniffed. Wiped my nose on the back of my hand. Waited.

"We're going to Bromley, lad," he said. I sniffed again. We, he'd said. We. I could feel my heart banging out of my chest.

"I know it's a long way away…" he said. Not as far as Australia, I thought.

"And I know you won't know anyone at first…" he said. I will, I thought, I'll know you.

"And it might be hard to leave all your old friends…" he said. It will be, I thought, but I'd still have a family.

"But there's the chance of a permanent stall, on the six-day market, and I know people down there from before – when I was a seaman – and it might be easier to get along, now that, you know…" He trailed off, looking around the kitchen again as though Mam might walk in at any time and he'd catch her with his arm round her waist and she'd lean into him with a smile. I swallowed over a lump in my throat and a funny noise came out.

"Is that a yes?" he said, and he actually looked nervous, like I might say no.

I nodded and he let out a breath, slowly.

"You and me, Ernie. We've got to stick together now, eh, lad?" He ruffled my hair, and caught me on the top of my stupid ear where it stuck out and even though it hurt it a bit it made my heart ache inside my chest. But in a nice way for once.

Two days later, after saying goodbye to Billy Sankey and handing the key back to Mr Gibbons, the landlord, I got on the back of Libby and Alf handed me my very own open-face helmet. I pulled it down, pinning my ears to my head, and he showed me how to strap it under my chin.

"Never ride without a helmet, Ernie," he said. "Promise?"

"Promise."

The neighbours waved as we puttered down the cobbles. Mrs Sankey wiped her eyes. She missed Mam, almost as much as we did. At the corner, Alf turned to me and said above the noise of Libby's engine, "Hold on tight, son."

And I did.

The Everyday

The shop was well laid out, the stock fully faced up. All product labels pointing towards the customer, all bottles and cans straight on the shelves. I nodded in approval even as the door swung shut behind me, bell jangling.

"What you two doing here?" Sue said from behind the counter.

"More like what you doing behind there?" I said. Alf wouldn't be happy, her messing about behind the cash desk. Sue ignored my question and looked to her mum. Charming.

"On our way to the lunch club," Phyllis said and my stomach rumbled loud enough for them both to look at me. Sue laughed. Phyl went over to the counter and they started chatting.

I walked off along the row of vegetables to check the produce. Long stems of rhubarb pink to white, next to the dark green heads of broccoli, the bright orange of baby carrots. I tucked in a couple of deep purple beetroot as they hung out of their box, inspected the potatoes for bruises or holes. The smell of earth and leaves filled my nostrils. It was a good smell.

The fruit side of the shop was just as colourful. Lemons, grapes, grapefruit, kiwis. Some fruit Alf wouldn't recognise, and I wouldn't know what to do with. I glanced out the back door of the shop. Was he out back?

"Looking okay, do you think, Dad?" Sue touched my arm.

"Looking great, Sue," I said. She beamed. Like I'd given her a present.

"What about the flowers, Dad?" She pointed at the corner, where she had a few bunches of daffs, a bucket of blue flowers and a big spray of white stuff.

"Hmm," I said.

"Customers love it, Dad," Sue said. "It's all extra."

I nodded.

"It's a decent shop," I said, turning in a small circle. She looked round with me, pleased.

"Hasn't really changed that much, has it?" she said. "In all this time."

"Over fifty years," said Phyllis. "Can you believe it?"

I frowned. "We used to dig these," I said, lifting a potato from the display. "Down the allotment." I rubbed the dusty dirt between my fingers.

"I know, Dad."

"And these," I said, picking up a red tomato and polishing it on my chest. "From the greenhouse."

"Yep," Sue said with a smile.

"Just to top up, you know. In case the wholesalers were short."

"The speciality tomatoes were the best seller this week," Sue said, pointing at punnets filled with all sorts. Little ones the size of marbles, big plum ones the size of a fist. Yellow ones, red ones, even green ones.

"They're not ripe," I said, frowning. She laughed.

"People pay good money for those, Dad," she said. There was a paper sign in front of the punnets with some numbers on it, which she seemed excited about. The bell tinkled.

"Well I never, how are you doing, Ernie?" a woman said too loudly next to me. "How nice to see you!" She must think I was deaf or something, the way she was bellowing at me.

I stared at her and then made myself smile. She had a big nose and a hair sticking out of her chin.

"Hi there, Mrs Mac," Sue said. "Mum and Dad just popped in on their way to lunch club."

The woman smiled and her chin hair waved up and down.

"We miss you at the darts club, Ernie. It's not the same without you on the team."

I wasn't sure what she wanted me to say to that, so I pretended to throw a dart in the air and everyone laughed.

"You always were a good player," the woman said. "Come down and see us some time."

Phyllis put her hand on my arm. She wanted to go. I could always tell when she wanted to go.

"We might just do that, Marion," she said. "When he's having a good day." All the women looked at each other.

"It's always a good day for darts," I said, picking up a strawberry off the top of the closest punnet and putting it in my mouth.

"Dad!" Sue said, rolling her eyes.

"Come on, love," said Phyl, steering me away from the woman. Maybe she didn't like her. She didn't seem to want to talk to her much. "Better go."

I glanced at the back door again. "Say bye to Alf," I said to Susie.

She bit her lip as she waved, but said she would. Phyllis opened the door and I followed her out.

Nina

Mr Browning, the college principal, looked as if he was trying to do that face where he is understanding but firm at the same time. The one that suggests he wants to empathise but his hands are tied. The one that tells Nina that, although he recognises she has problems with concentration, her work (or lack of it) is not good enough for college. She could only sit and wait for him to say the words.

Her mum's beetroot-stained hands twisted in her lap. Maybe, after all, she felt a little bit like Nina, who was kicking her feet frantically under the chair. Her mum nudged her with an elbow and she tried to stop, but very soon the rhythm started again from right inside her, until it got all the way to her toes and then they just had to tap.

"So, I'm sorry to say we've come to the end of the road here." Mr Browning leaned back in his chair and put his hands together on the desk, as though closing a sermon.

"You can't give her another chance?" Mum said and Nina's stomach dropped at the pleading in her voice. Please don't beg for me, she thought. "Nina told me she just needs a bit of help to get on top of things."

Mr Browning steepled his fingers and looked towards them.

Mum ploughed on. "It's so different from school, you see. She just needs help in scheduling the homework to help her prioritise things properly."

Nina felt the weight of not being able to cope with the everyday stuff that everyone else seemed to be able to do without a problem. It sat heavily on her. It felt like failure.

"She's already been allocated extra tutor time, Mrs Jackson. But she's only made it to the sessions once."

They both turned to Nina.

"He gave me *extra* stuff to do – a plan or something that he wanted me to pull together – which I only got half-finished and then I couldn't go back after that because I hadn't done it," she blurted. It was like everything else in her life, half done, half forgotten, totally screwed up.

"What about a mentor? Nina said she'd applied for one of those. That could help her?" Sue said, tapping her finger on the desk.

Nina held her breath, knowing what was coming next.

Mr Browning consulted a file on the table. "Nina was appointed a mentor last month, Mrs Jackson, a student in Year 13."

"And did that help, love?" Sue turned towards her daughter.

The headmaster cleared his throat and answered for her. "The student mentor said Nina left halfway through the first session because she 'had to buy chewing gum' and never came back."

Nina sighed. It was true. She really *had* needed chewing gum. It gave her jaw something to do and sometimes that helped her listen better. So, she thought it would help her to take in more of what the student mentor, Eliyah, was saying. She was *trying* to concentrate, because she could see that Eliyah, who studied maths and physics and chemistry, obviously had enough brains for both of them. The thing was, she popped out to buy the chewing gum, turned left out of the shop on autopilot and then only remembered she'd not gone back when she was halfway home. She'd been so embarrassed she left Eliyah sitting there on her own that she couldn't bring herself to go to the second session either, and after that had slunk round corners and hidden in classrooms if she ever saw her in the distance on campus.

Her mum let out a long, shaky breath and Nina dropped her head, not wanting to see her face.

"So, are there *no* other options?" Mum asked and Nina fizzed so fiercely inside that she had to grip the sides of the chair until her hands went white.

"Not to continue on this course at this college," the principal said. Nina felt queasy. So, it was done. She'd actually screwed it up so badly that there was no going back. "We have been through the correct process and it's time to draw the matter to a close, I'm afraid," he added.

"I see," Sue said and Nina imagined the disappointment coming off her in waves.

"Really, it's limited here, unless there is another course that Nina would like to sign up for next year?" Mr Browning tapped his pen and Nina knew they were both looking at her.

She lifted her head and saw the hope in her mother's eyes. She could apply for something else. She could come back.

"Is there anything that you think might appeal, Nina? Bearing in mind, we are a very academic college." Mr Browning sounded like he was answering his own question.

Nina's brain had stopped. She looked one to the other, trying to consider courses. But all she could think was that she hated maths, English, geography, history, French and all the sciences. She honestly couldn't think of any others. Her eyes were going dry with effort and she blinked and shook her head.

Her mum's shoulders lowered in defeat.

"What do we do next then?" she said softly.

"Well, it's law for young people to be in education until they are eighteen, Mrs Jackson," Mr Browning said. "But education comes in all shapes and sizes. So it might be worth looking at trades colleges for an apprenticeship for next year? Maybe beauty work, or hairdressing?"

Even as he said it, he looked like he knew he'd made a mistake. Who on earth was going to trust someone who couldn't keep their hands still with a pair of scissors near their ears or a wax strip on their undercarriage?

After that it was just the niceties. Her mum thanking him for telling her that he was kicking her daughter out of college and him saying good luck for the future.

But Nina didn't think she had one of those. She'd never heard of anyone being kicked out for failing college within two terms of starting. In fact she'd never heard of anyone being kicked out at all. Her chair scraped the wooden floor loudly as she stood up and faced her principal with his hand outstretched to her. She shook it. And the deal was sealed. She was the biggest failure she knew.

They crossed the college car park in silence. Nina wanted Sue to say something but was scared of what might come out.

But Sue said nothing until they were both in the car. She put the key in the ignition but then let her hands fall to her lap without turning it on. A few spots of rain hit the windscreen.

"I'm sorry, Mum," Nina whispered to fill the silence. "I'm really sorry."

Her mum's face watching the rain get harder made it worse. Nina thought she was trying not to cry.

"I really tried, Mum," Nina said then, louder than she intended, now angry with herself, her mum, Mr Browning. The fizzing was back and she wanted to throw open the car door, to run home, to feel some air on her face. Instead she banged the fingers of one hand into the palm of the other with a sharp pat, pat, pat, pat, pat.

"I know you did, love. But maybe you should have rethought the medication option. It might have helped."

Nina shook her head. "I told you, I don't want to take a pill every day of my life to 'fit in'. I want to be okay as I am."

They stared at each other and her mum seemed sad enough to break Nina's heart.

"I'm just rubbish," Nina said and it came out in a gulp. For God's sake. She mustn't cry.

Instead Mum pulled her over into a hug. "No, you're not," she said, squeezing her so hard that the handbrake stuck in Nina's side. "Don't say that, love. Nobody thinks you're rubbish in any way. I certainly don't think that, and nor does your dad." She squeezed her. "And I'm sure your fella doesn't think that either."

Nina blinked, remembering the last time she'd seen him, when he stopped kicking a can along the corridor to give her a thumbs-up to the jeers of his mates. "College isn't for everyone," Sue carried on, her voice muffled against Nina's hair. "Just remember Jeremy Clarkson…"

Nina sat back, so that she could see her mum's face.

"Pops said to me that he thinks I just haven't found my passion yet." Nina tugged at her mum's sleeve to make her point. She needed her mum to believe it. She needed to believe it herself.

That she wasn't the biggest idiot she knew. That she could still make her mum proud of her in some way. Her mum sighed as discreetly as she could and then smiled, resolutely.

"Well, at least we've got a plan B," she said, which was the first Nina had heard of it. Her mum turned the key in the ignition and the car headlights shone through the downpour.

"You can work with me in the shop, and we'll see if the trades college does an apprenticeship in retail. Lucky we've got a family business, eh?"

Nina's heart sank.

It was official.

She was a loser.

The Far Away

1957

Phyllis was not meant for me. Not originally. Or so she thought. I had different ideas from the outset.

The first time I set eyes on her, I was working on the stall on a Saturday, the busiest day of the week, before I'd got called up for my national service. I'd have been about seventeen. It was a dry day and the market was busy but sociable. Nobody scurried like they did when it rained. Everyone had time for a chat, a few minutes to pass before they went on their way. Our normal pitch, on the road between Tanner and Merrick, was smack in the middle of a long stretch of stalls, lining both sides of the street. The traders faced each other, watched each other's wares, minding each other's business. Budgie Jones was next to us with his stall of caged birds. The sound of canaries was as much a part of the market to me as Alf's patter. The other side was Jack Silver and his cutlery, and we faced onto Estrella the Spain and her linens. Tablecloths, napkins, the like. We all got on pretty well apart from the day one of Budgie's birds escaped the little stall cage and messed on Estrella's sheets.

Alf's height gave him the advantage on the market. He'd spot Mrs Hinch before she even reached the fish stall on the corner, and by the time she got to us he'd be greeting her with her usual veggies all bagged up. Or he'd recognise Mrs Green's scarf, the one with swirls on it she always tied tightly under her chin, and he'd be polishing an apple for her as she approached. Special promotion he'd say, with a wink, or "Got your name on them, these have". Rarely did they get away without buying. Apart from Nancy Shivers. She always went away with a few things. A bundle of carrots "that are on the way out" or a potato or two "with eyes in the back of their head". But she never put any money in his hand. He always folded her hand up and pushed it back at her. "Get out of here," he'd say. And off she'd go with a straggle of kids toddling behind that now had something to eat for their tea.

Alf's boy. That's who I was by then. I liked it. Belonging to him.

After the long journey on Libby to London, when I wasn't sure if I belonged to anyone, my legs wouldn't walk properly for days but I made sure never to be more than a stride behind him, just in case he lost me somewhere. Or left me behind accidentally. I worried he'd forget I was his now. But over the days, every time we stopped to talk to someone he recognised, or met someone new, he'd put his hand on my shoulder and eventually I realised Alf liked to feel me there too, just like I did him. He got us lodgings where I slept on a sofa and he snored magnificently while sleeping diagonally on a bed too short for him and then he set about getting his pitch at the market, promised as it was by an old navy friend of his.

We'd turned up together, him and I, setting out our stall on the first day. Me helping out early before my first day in a new class, a new school. Where I was the new boy for the first time in my life and called Ernie Ears from the off as there was another Ernie in the school and he had the normal-sized ears on the sides of his head. Where they all spoke different and laughed when I said "bath" instead of "barf" and "grass" instead of "grarse". It didn't last long though. I kept my head – and ears – down in school until the novelty wore off and after a bit I found some of the kids were nice and I made some new friends, though I still wished Billy Sankey was living next door.

But it was weird how soon Divine Street seemed a lifetime ago. We'd made a new one, just Alf and I. I still lingered outside the baker to smell the dough and close my eyes. And sometimes I imagined little fingers clutching mine and felt funny when I thought of Dot never growing up. But Alf was tall and loud, and there – and that made things better.

The early starts were harder in winter. Alf would be up and off to the wholesalers. He had a trailer-type cart he could attach to the back of Libby and he'd stock up on what we needed. I'd roll out the stall and start setting out. By the time he came back, it would be almost time for school. On Saturdays, I'd work all day and the other traders would wave or call at me as they went past.

"Go get your dad," they'd say to me, or "Tell your dad there's a pint behind the bar." I never corrected them. And nor did he. He'd give me a shove on the shoulder that fair heaved me off my feet, or a nudge with an elbow that felt like a spade. And he'd grin about it. "You're my boy now," he said once with a smile.

This one Saturday in September, when I saw Phyllis for the first time, I'd just finished school for good. Glad to be out of there as I'd been hanging on by my fingernails – maths and English were never my strong points. I much preferred being at the market, where I could handle the simple arithmetic and leave the patter to the professionals. The market rang with it. The calls, the prices. Puppies on sale one weekend, kittens the next. The queues of dirty-faced kiddies lined up at the sweet stand with their pennies in clammy hands. I felt at home there, standing next to Alf. I filled the bags and cleared the rubbish. He did the talking and pulled in the punters. At the end of the day, we packed up together and went home tired. It was about midday and my stomach was starting to tell me it was lunchtime. I couldn't wait to hear the church clock chime so that Alf would give me some coins to go and find a pie for us, or maybe a pasty.

And then I saw her.

A girl in a pink dress that pinched her in at the middle. Her hair in a ponytail, low at her neck. Swinging her bag as she walked, straight down the middle of the market. A couple of other girls walked with her, wearing similar clothes but not wearing them like she did. Two of them giggled behind their fingers as though they'd just heard a joke. She just walked, slightly to the side of them, part of the pack. She was the kind of girl that made my tongue stick to the roof of my mouth, and I prayed she didn't look my way.

"All right, girls," Alf called and I wanted to die, even though he said it a million times a day. The two at the back giggled again as if he'd said something funny. I edged behind the stall, so as not to be seen.

"Want something to sweeten your day, sweetheart?" Alf was saying, making my neck get hot. Please don't let her look over.

"You lot look fresh as peaches yourselves," Alf called. They were level with us now, close enough for discomfort. She was quite tall, for a girl.

"Here you go girls, sweet treats for you." Alf picked a juicy tangerine from the stall and tossed it in the air towards them.

The friends gasped and flapped their hands, unsure as to what to do. The girl simply shot a hand upwards and caught it above her head without hesitation and without fear of dropping it. It made a satisfying sound, steady and sure.

The girls all clapped and pretended to sigh in relief that it had been caught. When in actual fact it had never been in doubt. She wouldn't have dropped it for the world.

The trio started to move on. And the tall girl with laughing eyes held the tangerine in her palm and smiled, full face, at Alf.

"Thanks, Mister," she said.

My heart went bang.

The Everyday

Phyllis is unbuttoning the front of my pyjamas and the cold air of the bathroom is rushing in to the gaps.

"Brrr," I mutter and shake myself.

"Keep yourself still Ernie, won't you?" She's got a little line between her eyebrows where she's focusing on my buttons and she doesn't even raise her eyes to look at me. Whatever she's doing, she's determined. She's always been like that, Phyl. The little line started years ago with her knitting baby blankets in front of the television, or frowning at socks as she darned them, or sewing on those little name tapes that Stephen and Susan had to have in their uniforms. It's just got deeper and deeper over the years. How many years has it taken so far? For it to always be there now and not come and go.

She undoes another button and I shift one foot to another on the tiled floor. My feet are cold too. I glance down at them and there they are, sticking out of the bottom of my pyjama trousers, white-looking, horny old nails.

"Well, if you won't do it yourself..." she says. Her voice is light, as though she's joking, but the way that she's tugging at my clothes shows she means business. "I'll just have to help you, won't I?"

"What are you doing, woman?" I try to pull the edges of my pyjama top together, keeping out the air as it creeps onto my skin. I want to put on a pullover, go and sit in the chair. The bathroom light above me hums. It reminds me of the hospital. I step backwards but my back is against the wall.

"Just going to have a shower, Ernie," Phyllis says. I snort.

"Why?" I say. "Is it Sunday?"

She laughs then, outright, and the little line disappears. I see my Phyl. The one that loves budgerigars and fountains. A flicker of relief licks my tummy, which has been feeling tight and sore.

"We don't just get clean on a Sunday, you silly old goat," she says, wiping the last of her laugh away on the back of her hand. "It's not the seventies any more, you know."

"Who you calling an old goat?" I say and try to pull my pyjamas together again while she's still smiling. But it doesn't work.

"You." She pushes at my chest and gets to work on the next button. She's not giving up. In one movement she slips the top off my shoulders and down my arms. My skin puckers and moves of its own accord. "Doctor says it's important to keep clean."

"Brrr," I say again and wrap my arms round myself.

"It'll be warm in there," she says and nods towards the corner. There's a see-through box. Floor to ceiling. Something prickles inside. Why does she want to put me in a box?

She puts her hands on my waistband and I clamp mine over hers, scared.

"Come on silly," she says and her voice has that tone to it again. Like it's light, but I know it's not. It's like wire underneath. I want her to stop. I want her to put the kettle on and sit in the chair next to mine.

"It won't take long," she says, and it sounds like she's got her teeth gritted. Like when she scrubs the kitchen floor. She sounds mean. I don't like this Phyllis. I want the other one back.

She's pushing my trousers down and I'm holding onto her hands to keep them up. She's strong these days though and she's winning. I can feel the air moving down my body as she makes me almost naked. The light is humming. The tiles are cold on my feet. The draught from the door is making the hairs stand up on my arms. I don't like the way I feel inside. It's like when Mammy died. Something moving in my guts.

"There we go," she says as finally my trousers hit the floor and she takes my hands and helps me step out of them. She opens the see-through door and turns a silver lever. Water starts spurting from the top and she's got her hand in it, waving it about.

"Get it to the right temperature for you, my love," she's saying and it's like she's all happy now and I'm wondering what's next. Will she put me in a nice warm jumper and a pair of trousers? She wipes her hand on a towel hanging beside me on a bar and smiles again.

"In you go, then," she says, moving herself out of the way. In where? Is it time to go and sit in my chair?

She takes my hand and I feel better, just for a moment, but then she's tugging me towards the box, gently but definitely like she wants me to get in there.

I don't want to go in but I don't know what else to do. She helps me step in onto a white floor.

"Careful, now, love," she says. "It's slippery."

I look down and she pushes me further in. Things are suddenly hitting my head. Tiny little pings and taps, running down my face, into my ears. I cover my eyes, rub at them blindly. The water is running all over me, coursing down my back, running into bits of me that are normally warm and dry. My eyes won't open properly and I can't see Phyllis. I reach my hands out for her but she's not there. I can hear a funny noise and realise it's me.

"Just rub yourself down, Ernie," she says. "Come on, love." She's pushing something into my hand – a sponge. Like the one I used to wash the car with. When she made me get the saloon. I look at it and try to take a step out the door but she's having none of it.

"Just got to get clean, Ern." She's got my hand with the sponge in it and she's rubbing it on my tummy, under my arms.

"Stop." I try to push her away but she's got the sponge herself now and it's under my other arm, burrowing like a terrier looking for rats in Divine Street.

I want to get out. I want her to stop.

Now she's fussing down there. Rubbing at me and I try to push her hand away. What on God's earth is happening?

"Don't want an infection, do we, love?"

It's like she used to do with Stephen in front of the sink when he was a boy. But that was because he was dirty. And little. And couldn't do it himself. What's she doing it for me for?

I grab her arm, right on the squishy bit, and hold on. I squeeze it so tight I can feel my teeth clench. She makes a squeal and stumbles slightly and I can see the sleeve of her cardigan getting wet under the spray. Just like me.

"All done," she says suddenly and there's a smile, like she's just seen a rainbow over the sea. She fiddles with the silver lever behind me and the pins and needles on my head stop. And the air rushes in again and my skin turns to bumps all over.

She holds my hands again and lets me step out. I can hear what's left of my teeth chattering and my face feels shaky.

"Brrr," I say and she laughs.

"Is that all you've got to say for yourself today, Ern?" She wraps me in a towel and pulls me towards her and suddenly I feel my eyes get hot and wet and I feel like I couldn't speak even if I wanted to. Not with this big lump in my throat. I try to clear it and she starts to rub me, briskly, making my skin pink and dry. It reminds me of Susan, fresh from the bath on a Sunday, watching TV on the sofa before bed. Her pink cheeks. The smell of the soap.

Soon she's got me in new clothes. A shirt she says matches my eyes. A big warm jumper. She even kneels down and stuffs my feet into a pair of slippers. I look at her head while she's down there. She's got very white, Phyl has. But I think it probably best not to mention it. She doesn't like to think she's getting old.

The TV is on and now I'm in my chair.

"Turn it up," I say and it gets louder as Phyl presses something. There's a woman on there complaining about her neighbour.

"Who knitted her face and dropped a stitch?" I ask, but Phyl is stretching out her back, rolling her shoulders in the chair.

"Look at the state you've got me in," Phyllis is saying and showing me her arms and one of her arms has a patch of redness as if she's knocked it. Her sleeves are wet right up to the shoulders. Her cheeks are pink too. Whatever she's been doing, she's got herself in a right mess.

Nina

The other college couldn't take Nina until September.

She'd missed too much of the current year to join and so had to wait for the new intake. Her heart had sunk as it meant that all the sixteen-year-olds in the year would think she was already weird for this, and that was before they discovered all the other oddities about her.

What were the chances of making friends now?

Sue had nodded along quite happily at the news though and said, "You can work in the shop full time then. It will give me a bit more time to help Nan with Pops," as though this was the perfect solution to everyone's lives.

Luckily it was one of the afternoons that Mum was at Nan's that motorbike boy rode past.

Nina was spinning round and around on the stool behind the counter while the shop was empty when she heard the waspy buzz of the engine with its telltale knocking noise and then spotted his white **SPLAT HAT** as he pulled onto the high street. He had a mate following him, on an old Lambretta, who putt-putted along in the rear. She checked her watch. College had just finished. They parked almost outside her shop and she held her breath as they swaggered into the newsagent opposite, Nina hearing the doorbell jangling loudly as they entered.

Two women entered the greengrocers, making its own smaller doorbell jingle. They strolled around the displays, chatting as they checked ripeness and filled their baskets. They arrived at the counter as the bell opposite jangled again, but a quick glance showed it was an elderly man with a pull-along basket that came out onto the pavement.

"How's your mum?" the women asked and Nina gave in to small talk as she weighed and bagged their produce. Making sure to double-check the numbers she pressed on the card machine so that she didn't overcharge them. Remembering to smile and be polite, as "the face of the shop" as Mum always reminded her.

"Tell Sue we were asking after her," one of the women said as she pulled open the door a couple of minutes later, and it was only then that Nina saw the boys standing directly outside her shop window, watching. They were right there on the pavement, with their hands cupping their faces to the window, staring at her with their noses pressed up against the glass. She jumped so much she nearly fell off her stool. It wobbled and she clutched at the counter to keep herself upright. They sniggered, then both took a long drag on their vapes and blew out endless plumes of haze. Nina knew she was bright red in the face. She stood quickly and walked to the rear of the shop and out of the back door, shut it and leaned against it in one movement.

She must have looked so stupid. God, it couldn't get any worse. Why couldn't she just have smiled and waved, like any normal person? She fanned her face and pulled at the neck of her t-shirt to cool herself down.

The doorbell jingled and she knew a customer had come in and she'd have to go out. She couldn't leave the shop empty. She just hoped the boys weren't outside any more.

Which in fact, they weren't. Because, when she opened the back door and stepped into the shop again, she could see very clearly that they were now INSIDE. Well, he was anyway. Motorbike boy. The one who always gave her a funny look. His mate was now over the road, tinkering with his Lambretta. Nina clapped her hands together in front of her three times for absolutely no reason at all, which surprised him, so she clenched her fists at her sides in a superhuman effort to hold them still.

"All right?" he asked.

She nodded. Then added "Yes" for good measure.

They looked at each other. He was taller than her. His hair was a bit greasy, from wearing a helmet, she supposed, and he slicked it back on his head with a palm.

"Been looking for you at college," he said. She nodded. Her tongue felt the size of a cow's, taking up every spare millimetre of space in her mouth. There was no room for words. He nodded around the shop. "Guess you're not there any more, then?"

She shook her head and then gave herself a mental kick. Say something. Idiot.

"Going to the trades college in September," she murmured. "Working here until then." And for the rest of my life, she thought but managed to keep that bit to herself.

He nodded, picked up a pomegranate and tossed it one hand to the other. On him it looked casual, but she knew if she picked anything up at the moment she'd be chucking it about like a circus juggler. She clenched her fists even tighter.

"They have up to a thousand seeds in them," she said, out of nowhere.

He grinned, put it back on the display and moved over to the strawberries.

"And they're not actually berries at all," she said, surprising herself.

He laughed then.

"You're like the fruit master," he said.

"I'm fruit-o-pedia," she said, wondering what exactly she was going on about.

He laughed again and she felt something inside her bubble. He thought she was funny. He sniffed loudly and stuck his thumbs in his belt loops.

"So, wanna go out sometime?"

"Yes," she blurted and clapped her hands three times again in front of her. Honestly, she'd seen less clapping in a gospel choir. What on earth was she doing?

He looked a bit startled but nodded. "What time do you finish tomorrow?"

She made herself lean – nonchalantly, she thought to herself – on the counter before answering. This was to make sure her flappy hands behaved themselves.

"Five," she said.

"I'll be back, then." He lowered his chin and stared at her intently. She froze. It was that look again. The one that made her think he liked her. She stared back at him, not sure what to do or say. Finally, he nodded as if he'd given her a telepathic message and turned towards the door.

She let her shoulders slump in relief but then jolted upright as though she'd been electrocuted when he turned back towards her.

"What's your name then?" he said. "You're not really called Birdie, are you?"

Oh GOD. Mortifying. "Nina," she managed to get out.

"You probably know mine," he said with a smirk.

"Errr, no," Nina answered with a hint of embarrassment. Should she?

"Taylor," he said, his thumb towards his chest, "Taylor Jenkins." He pulled his mobile from his pocket. "Gonna give me your digits?"

Nina stared at him stupidly for a moment before realising what he meant. Then she reached for his phone and tapped her number in. He sent an immediate text and she heard her own phone beep in the desk drawer.

"That's mine," he said and she wondered what he'd typed so quickly. "Laters." And he pulled open the door a bit too energetically, making the bell jingle almost off the hook.

She watched him swagger over the road to his mate. They exchanged a few words and then his mate gave him a dead arm, it looked like.

Nina picked up a lime from the display as she watched them both mount their motorbikes and zigzag dangerously up the high street. Someone beeped at them as they went round the corner.

"Now you've got my number, you can call me any lime," she said to herself.

After that first text, which said "hello" – rather unimaginatively, thought Nina, but then kicked herself because what would *she* have thought of to write so fast herself – there was nothing else until she was almost asleep that night. The ping of her phone dragged her back to her bedroom and she rubbed her eyes and sat up in bed. Nobody ever texted her, unless it was Mum, and she was asleep next door. Or Jess, but that would be daytime too, checking on her or asking her to come and babysit the kids before she pulled her last remaining hair out. But the name on the screen was Taylor and she stared at it wide-eyed, the phone illuminated in the dark of her room.

Of course, she thought, he would be texting now to say "Ha, only joking!" She held her breath and pressed her lips together, opened the message.

"See you tomorrow."

She held the phone with both hands as though it might explode and read it again. In fact, she read the three words at least ten times before she breathed out.

See you tomorrow. That meant he was still coming. And that he was looking forward to it because he was confirming it. She shut her eyes tight and opened her mouth wide in a silent scream and pummelled the bed either side of her for a few seconds before looking at it again.

He was thinking of her. Now. At this minute. Late at night. She checked the time. At 11.47p.m. on a Wednesday night, Taylor Jenkins was thinking of her.

She grinned and threw herself back on her pillow.

Oh God, wait, that meant he might still be thinking of her *now* and waiting for her to reply. She racked her brains for something interesting to reply, or funny, or, better still, intriguing. Her mind flicked through random thoughts – rabbits and carrot jokes and cappuccino with sprinkles on – none of it helpful. She breathed out and finally tapped a response. One symbol. Not even a word. A smiley face. It would have to do. Then she pressed send and it whizzed off to wherever Taylor Jenkins was.

It took her ages to get to sleep afterwards, wondering if he might send something else. This boy who thought about her late at night. She'd never known anyone to like her enough to think her about her at all, let alone when they should be asleep, and Nina decided she quite liked it.

Mum did a double-take in the morning when Nina came down the stairs and she wondered if she'd overdone the mascara. She ducked her chin but Mum just gave her a squeeze and said, "You look nice today, love" as she opened the door for them to head out.

It was only when they reached the shop and Nina took off her coat, releasing the liberal spritz of perfume she'd applied that morning, that Mum asked what the special occasion was. Nina had an overwhelming urge to laugh and a giggle escaped. Mum laughed too, although slightly nervously, so Nina explained, "I've got a date this afternoon."

A ripple passed over Sue's face, which erupted into a massive grin and a nudge.

"The one from college?" she said, pulling her apron over her head and tying it behind her back.

Nina nodded.

"Well, what's he called?"

"Taylor," Nina said and finished his name with a smile.

Sue did an elongated oooooooo as if Taylor was the most fancy name in the world, but Nina didn't mind.

"What's he like?" asked Sue, turning on the cash till and then heading out back to flick the switch on the kettle.

"I don't know really," Nina said, and then told what she knew. "He's still at college. He said he's been looking for me there."

"You haven't spoken much yet?"

"Not yet."

"So what do you like about him then?" Sue asked, head on one side. "I bet he's funny. I imagine you having a nice, funny, kind boyfriend. Like you."

Nina paused. Was Taylor funny? Or nice? Or kind? She'd only seen him throwing chips about and taking the mickey out of Pops. Neither of which seemed to fit into those categories. She shook her head, remembering the way he looked at her. Nobody else looked at her like that.

"I don't know him very well yet." She stood on one leg and spun round, and, when she stopped and faced her mother again, finished her sentence with a bright red face. "But I know that he likes me."

Sue's face shadowed and she opened her mouth to say something, but the doorbell jingled and she had to serve an old lady instead.

And after that, there was an early-morning rush, so it wasn't until ten thirty that they got their first cup of tea. Then Mum threw a curveball into Nina's day. In fact, not anything as small as a curveball.

Sue threw a grenade into the plan, when she announced with delight, after a quick consultation via text message, that Nan didn't need her that afternoon and she'd be staying at the shop. So she could check Taylor out for herself.

Nina heard the telltale knocking of the black motorbike at last at 5.19p.m. For the past nineteen minutes she'd been jigging foot to foot and trying not to look out of the shop window at the high street.

Sue had already asked her three times if she was sure he was coming at five o'clock and checked her watch about a million times, the last few times with a little sigh. Nina couldn't tell if this was because she wanted to go home for her dinner but didn't want to miss the chance to gawp at Taylor, or because she was making some commentary on his timekeeping. Probably both. When she heard the motorbike at last she felt her insides relax and tense at the same time. He'd turned up as he'd promised.

She jumped up and down ten times on the spot, tiny and fast, to get rid of some energy and then went to open the door. Sue put both hands out in front of herself as though patting the air flat, telling her to calm down.

Fat chance.

Taylor strolled in and then did his own double-take when he saw Sue there too, pulling on her coat.

"Don't worry, Mum's not coming too! She's on her way home," Nina said and he snorted a laugh. She grinned. He still thought she was funny then. Off to a good start.

"Hi, Taylor," Mum said. "I'm Sue." She smiled kindly at him and Nina felt a weird pride inside that made her chest feel full.

"All right?" Taylor said, which Nina didn't think the most appropriate of replies, but Mum took it in her stride and used her "happy to meet you" voice again. "I'm fine, thanks. Have you had a good day at college?"

"Ha!" He snorted. "That's a good one!" Nina felt her stomach getting tighter, not sure this was going in the right direction.

"Oh, do you not enjoy your course?" Mum, still smiling, locked the cash till and put the key in her bag.

"Waste of time, really," Taylor said, and Nina looked at him with as much interest as Mum, to see what he'd say next. This was all news to her. "I'm going to be famous on social media, TikTok or YouTube or whatever, and so I don't really need college."

Nina had shown her mum different films on TikTok, dance routines and funny animals, so Mum knew what he was talking about. But Nina saw her look at Taylor now to see which of these categories he might be famous in.

"Are you a dancer then?" she asked and he snorted again, making Nina take a step back out of the spray range.

"No, but I've already got almost a hundred followers. My last video of doing a wheelie got over a thousand views."

Mum said, "Wow" with a little whistle but it didn't sound very sincere and Nina jigged foot to foot, wishing she'd asked Taylor all this stuff on her own.

"Shall we go?" she said to Taylor and he seemed happy to oblige. Although she was feeling like it might not be such a good idea after all.

"What are you two up to then?" Mum said as they opened the shop door and the bell jingled with more optimism than Nina felt.

"Burger?" Taylor said with a raised eyebrow at Nina. She agreed, not having given any actual thought to what they would do if he actually turned up.

"I got you an extra helmet," he said, nodding towards the motorbike parked opposite. There was a blue open-visor helmet sitting next to the SPLAT HAT on the saddle. A shot of excitement bolted through Nina for the first time since he'd started talking, which Mum squashed as quickly as it appeared.

"You're not going on that motorbike."

Nina shot a look at her in disbelief. What was she doing? Why would she embarrass her like that in front of Taylor? After she'd just been nice to him?

"It'll be fine, Mum," she said, widening her eyes at her in a silent plea to back off.

"No way, Nina. Motorbikes aren't safe." Sue locked the shop door behind her.

"Pops always had one!" Nina dared not look at Taylor and could feel the rush of blood colouring her neck.

"No," Mum said firmly. Then she turned to Taylor and said, "Just in case you got the urge to pull another wheelie."

Nina looked at him, mentally urging him to say something to put Mum's mind at rest.

"You might have a point there, Sue," he said in a way that Nina couldn't interpret. "You never know when the urge might strike."

Nina felt something inside her deflate and realised it was her dreams.

But she was determined not to let her mum think she knew best when it came to boyfriends.

Nina nudged Taylor and together they walked off up the road towards McDonald's and a burger she didn't really want to eat.

The Far Away

1958

The next time I saw the girl in the pink dress was the day I finally took my motorcycle test. I'd wanted to take it for a year, but Alf had held me off.

"No rush, boy. We don't want Libby getting hurt now, do we?" He'd laughed but I knew it wasn't just Libby he was worried about.

He said if I was going to ride motorbikes I had to know how to maintain one first and over the summer he spent every spare hour showing me how to grease, take apart, flush out and put Libby back together to keep her in perfect running order.

Finally, he gave in. On the promise I'd always wear a helmet, whether or not this hurt my ears, which, despite my wishes, had not got better with age. I swore and he held out the keys to Libby, and I had to stop my hand from shaking as I took them.

He taught me well.

To respect my bike. To respect the road. To respect the weather.

He taught me to look twice for dangers – for potholes that might throw me off, or cars that might open their doors as I passed and knock me flying. He pointed out chevrons and bollards and took me out in rain and in darkness, teaching me how to drive by the single headlight showing the way. Now that I knew how to look after the bike, he made very sure I knew how to look after myself on it.

I was ready. I had to meet the tester at a car park in Bromley. Alf watched me from the kerb as I pulled away and just before I turned the corner I glanced back at him in my mirror. He stood with his head back, looking at the sky for a moment as though asking something, or making a wish.

I took a left under the arches and Libby felt smooth and steady as I headed towards the high street. It was as I passed the butcher's that I saw the three girls again. The same three that had been in the market. I recognised them straight away.

Phyllis straight and tall between the shorter girls. By then, I knew her name. Phyllis Marshall. Her father owned Marshall's shoe shop. Phyllis went to the local girls' school. The other girls were called Pat and Daphne, not that it mattered to me. It was only Phyllis I was interested in. I'd walked past the doorway to the shoe shop a hundred times in the past month hoping to catch a glimpse. Sometimes she'd be there, behind the counter, serving a customer, and I'd see her write studiously on the sales pad, the tip of her tongue edging from the corner of her mouth.

And now she was going to see me on Libby. Not just as the boy at the market. The one that stacked fruit and lugged boxes about. But one who could ride a motorbike. Who had transport. A man. I sat up slightly straighter as I approached. I slowed, to allow a car to pull out and I was almost alongside them. They looked at me. All three of them. Phyllis's eyebrows were perfect arches.

Ignoring thoughts of Alf and his warnings of distractions and dangers, I took my right hand off the handlebar and held it up in a wave. Her eyebrows went higher but a tiny curve of a smile lifted the corners of her mouth. And then I was past and I put my hand back on the grips with relief and a heart that beat right into my helmet.

She'd seen me. She knew I was alive.

The actual test itself seemed less worrying after that. If I could wave at Phyllis Marshall, I could do anything.

I drove the test route without fault and answered the questions, and was then certified to ride a motorbike on my own. Something I'd dreamed about ever since Libby came into my life. On the way back home to Alf, I got to thinking. If I hadn't seen her, would I have failed? Was it an omen that I saw her again on that day? Was she my lucky charm?

By the time I opened the door at home, beaming literally ear to ear, I was ready to run back to Marshall's and ask her out. Maybe a walk on the Sunday would be a good start.

But Alf was waiting there for me, with an envelope in his hands, my name typed on the front and the Queen's crest. My call-up for national service.

And my life changed all over again.

Two weeks later I'd be gone. It was "no time to be courting", Alf said, or even thinking about it. But as I passed Marshall's Shoes, I saw Phyllis a few more times through the doorway and knew I had to at least make sure she knew who I was before I went. I needed just something to remember her by to keep me going.

The bell jangled as I pushed open the shop door, louder than my nerves as I stepped into the shop. It was the first time I'd been inside, seen the rows of shoes shiny in the afternoon light, the smell of leather heavy in the air. I was the only customer as, having lurked outside on the corner for ten minutes, I'd timed it just right. I quickly saw the shop was divided, women's on one side, men's on the other, with a mending station in the corner for heels and soles that needed replacing.

I stepped quickly towards the men's shelves and slicked my hair back over my forehead while I still had it, already dreading the short back and sides the army would cut for me when I arrived. Mr Marshall looked at me over his glasses from the counter and I swallowed best I could over the lump in my throat.

"Afternoon, young man," he said. "What can I help you with today?"

I turned towards the boots, desperate for a glimpse of her rather than a conversation with her father. "Thinking of some new shoes," I said, stupidly, buying for time.

"Well, you're in the right place," he said jovially and put his papers to one side as though he were preparing to step out to serve me.

Phyllis saved me just then by walking in from the back room, the storeroom maybe, or the kitchen, straight onto the shop floor. She was smoothing her hands down on her apron as she came in and her eyes widened – just a flash – when she saw me, and the faintest hint of colour crept in at her neck.

"Ah, Phyllis," her father said, "Will you help the young man?" and bent back to his books, frowning over his columns of numbers. Phyllis and I looked at each other, our eyes met and held, both like rabbits in the headlights of a car. It was exactly what I wanted and more than I could hope for, all in one. I wondered how men in the movies made it look so easy.

"Men's shoes?" she said. Her voice was low, like it came from the back of her throat. It wasn't high and giggly like the girls that travelled in packs through the market.

I nodded, again stupidly, and she pointed at the shelves beside me. I turned towards them, and she took a single step closer.

"Not sure what I'm looking for to be honest," I said, not sure how to start.

"Formal wear or everyday?" she asked and I shrugged, checking her dad was busy with his book before replying, more quietly.

"I don't really need either right now," I said and she cocked her head to one side in surprise. "I'm going off to do my service, see?"

"You going on your motorbike?" she said, and I felt a surge of something happy. Recognition. She knew who I was. She'd seen me on Libby.

"I wish!" I grinned. "It's my stepdad's."

Her face changed like maybe I'd lost a bit of credit.

"I'll get one of my own when I get back though."

She nodded as though she believed me. As though she thought I really would.

"When do you go then?" she asked, running her finger along the front of the shelves. She came up to about my chin. Her back was very straight and her hair was the darkest colour of the conkers we threaded and fought with in autumn.

"Tomorrow."

She pursed her lips to one side as though considering something and I racked my brains for something else to say. Something important. I had to make a mark somehow. Two years was a long time. What if she forgot about me?

Her father rustled his papers together and walked out into the back room. I knew this was my chance.

I picked up a boot from the row in front of me, turned it slowly in my hands. "I might not need shoes now, but it's good to know you've got everything I want for when I come back again."

She flicked her face at me, the flush at her neck almost reaching her chin now, and she bit her lip under her top teeth.

Her dad walked back in empty-handed, and raised a quizzical eye in our direction. I cleared my throat and she smoothed her apron again and I hoped to God she knew I was talking about more than just shoes.

"So I'll see you again, then," I said, placing the brown boot carefully back next to its partner. "When I get back."

"Good luck," she said with a little wave.

The Everyday

"Happy anniversary!" Everyone shouted and clapped and something went bang in the air beside me.

I clutched my heart like I'd been shot and staggered about a bit and everyone laughed as bits of coloured paper fell all around my face. Phyllis took my hand and pulled me next to her again and she smelled like roses. I picked a tiny bit of the paper from her hair where it rested and suddenly felt like I'd done it before. Everyone was cheering and there was music.

"Congratulations, and celebrations…" the music boomed out. Who'd put bloody Cliff Richard on? That was all we needed.

"Photo!" Sue stepped towards me out of the crowd. She had a dress on that was a bit low in the front if you asked me. "Get together!" She motioned to Phyl and me and everyone else stepped back to give us a bit of room. I felt like I was in a zoo, everyone staring.

I put my arm round Phyllis's shoulders and pulled her towards me. She always liked a cuddle, Phyl.

"Yay!" people were shouting, and "Congratulations!" Cliff was still going; I never did like him.

But I liked the way Phyl beamed at me. Even though I saw the powder on her face was sitting in her creases, I thought it best not to say. She'd be sad. But her smile was the same as it had always been. Right from when she caught the tangerine.

I grinned.

"You look nice," I said because she did and her smile got the biggest I'd seen it for ages.

"We did well, didn't we Ernie?" she said, putting a hand to my cheek. "Look at us. Who would have thought it?"

"Another photo, Mum!" Sue said and then pointed something at us.

"Where's her camera?" I said to Phyl and she laughed and nudged me before tucking her arm behind my back.

"You know them, everything on their phones nowadays. She'll send us the photos later."

The photos were over then apparently and there were loads of people round us.

Sue and Josh and Nina were right up front, Nina bouncing side to side.

"Happy anniversary, Dad," Sue said as she gave me a hug. Everyone seemed to want one today. Daisy was next, she had a dress on with a bow in the front. She didn't look too impressed with it and when I tugged at it she screwed up her face.

"I tried to pull it off," she whispered in my ear and I laughed.

"Should have tried harder," I said. She snorted out of her tiny snub nose and it reminded me of someone else.

Freddie had a tie on and he pulled at his collar every few minutes. I winked at him and he frowned and shrugged.

Mary from the bakery was there without her apron on, Mike from the butcher's wearing a suit like he was at a wedding. In fact, all the guests looked like they had their best clobber on. Including me. My suit almost buttoned up still but not quite. We'd had quite a laugh about it before we left the house. She'd said I could leave it open as I had a waistcoat underneath. Waistcoat! Me! Who would have thought it?

My hair was all smart too. Phyllis had wet it down with a brush and tidied it up. It felt nice, the bristles on my head.

"You scrub up well," said a woman with blue-black hair and a nose stud and lots of tattoos. No idea who she was, but I thanked her and told her she looked fantastic too. I pointed to the ink of an eagle that covered her whole shoulder, its wings spanning front to back.

"Like it?" she said and I nodded a yes, not sure how to say no.

"Pukka, ain't it?" She smiled and I saw that one of her teeth was gold. I wondered how much I'd get for it down the market.

"Proper party!" a man said to me, mouthing exaggeratedly, shaking my hand. I nodded, not sure where I knew him from. "Well deserved!"

"Thanks," I said, just for something to say.

"Lots of people don't get here, do they?" he said, pulling a different face.

"No," I agreed, wondering was there a problem with the buses if people couldn't get there.

"We're the lucky ones, aren't we mate?" he asked, and then he was gone. I turned to see where he was heading, but everyone else was talking to each other, deep in conversations with their backs to me. I was alone in the circle of people. I peered into the corners, watched the party. Wondered where Alf was. Probably propping up the bar somewhere. I'd find him in a bit.

There was a banner across the door of the room. Coloured balloons hung everywhere. They were pretty. Two extra-big numbers that floated alone on the stage.

I could see through to the bar of the Rose and Crown out of the door in the corner. The barman was polishing glasses with a white tea towel. My usual chair by the fire would be quite comfy about now and I wondered if I could go and have a sit-down. Perhaps Phyllis would come with me. Leave people to get on with their partying in peace. Where was she? I peered into the crowd, a knot in my belly.

When I spotted her I knew she wouldn't want a sit-down. She looked happy as she moved from person to person. She hugged people and kissed cheeks and laughed that tinkling laugh of hers that although I was too far away to hear I could still feel as I loved it so much. She was wearing her special earrings, the little tiny diamond ones she only took out of the box for special occasions. They glinted like glass in the light. She kept them so clean. So polished. I suddenly wanted her next to me. Just for a minute. To hold my hand.

The music changed again, thank God. No more Cliff. A man's voice on the next record, counting, "1, 2… a 1, 2, 3". Then a drumbeat kicked in. I knew that voice. Chris Montez. The introduction did something inside of me. And one of my feet started to tap.

I knew exactly what I wanted to do. I crossed the room to Phyllis and tapped her arm. She stopped mid-conversation with a woman and turned to me.

"Let's dance," I said, indicating the music. She cocked an ear, listening, just as Chris Montez sang exactly the same words.

"It is!" she said and laughed. "Fancy you remembering that!" She leaned slightly towards the woman. "This is the music from our courting days!"

The Everyday and Far Away

"No," I said, holding out my hand to her. "I mean us. Let's dance."

She hesitated for a split second, her eyebrow shooting up towards her hairline. Then she put her drink down on a nearby table and let me lead the way. I felt my spine straighten, my chin lift as I led my girl onto the dance floor.

Except it wasn't exactly a dance floor. More like a corner of the room with tiles instead of carpet. We stood facing each other in the middle and held both hands together, while we waited for a beat. Then we started.

My feet knew exactly what they were doing. I might shuffle around the house sometimes or creak when I sat down, but the music was everything and we were in it. I knew people were watching us and I didn't care. I knew what I was doing, and I wasn't worried. Phyl and I were good at dancing, we always had been. People would leave a little space around us at the dance hall, because they knew we spun, we moved, we took up room. The lights were flashing pink and blue and it made it hard to see as I pushed her back and then pulled her in to me again. But she went away, our arms stretched between us, and came back again exactly as she should. We did it again, turning as we did, her feet light as a girl's. She was the best partner I'd ever had, Phyllis. She turned, she twisted, she never missed my hand, she never lost a beat. I used to pick her up and throw her off again and she loved that. Her skirts used to fly, flashing her petticoats and sometimes even her stocking tops. The other girls used to watch, wishing they could dance like her. When I was dancing I never felt like I had big ears. I didn't feel like I had ears at all.

My blood was banging around my body and my face felt stretched around my smile when the music stopped and there was suddenly loads of clapping. A whole circle of people were around us, but when I looked they weren't the dance-hall crowd. No John Blackmore, or his brothers Jim and Bob. No slim young men with slicked hair and suits. These were old people. Grey or white hair. Some of them bald. Some who looked like they would not be able to jive if you held a gun to their head. And then some that looked too young to know what jiving was. Poor sods. But what I was feeling was the best feeling in the world.

"There's life in the old dog yet," I puffed to Phyllis, just like Alf used to say, as I held her hand to my own chest. She must be able to feel my heart against my ribs, the racket it was making.

Phyllis laughed and fanned her front with her hands. She was out of breath too but beaming.

"That was the best anniversary present ever," she said and gave me a kiss on the cheek.

"That was amazing!" someone called and she did a little curtsey and then pulled me towards her and I did a bow too and everyone cheered.

I thought it might be the most wonderful day of my life, and of Phyl's too, I hoped.

Nina

Everywhere she looked there was another white or bald head, some she recognised, had grown up with – old friends of her grandparents from the high street, or families of the stallies on the market. People they'd met along the way, at different points in their lives, all there to celebrate this huge anniversary with them. It was nice for them, to have a good turnout. Sue kept remarking what a milestone it was – to be fifty-five years married.

"Having fun, love?" Sue put an arm round Nina's shoulders, which immediately made her want to shrug it off. But she knew it would hurt her feelings so flicked her own thumb with her finger as quickly as she could instead and let the arm rest there.

"Uh-huh."

Her mum started swaying a bit, still holding on to her, and Nina's stomach contracted in terror. Don't say she was going to try to dance with her. She wouldn't do that, surely. Nobody else was even dancing since Nan and Pops stopped, apart from her niece Daisy. And Daisy was only a very young girl. Nina planted her feet as solidly as she could to stop herself rocking with her mum and looked around for a distraction. No way was she dancing to Cliff Bloody Richard or whoever it was.

"What's the food like?" she asked quickly and her mum glanced over at the buffet, still holding on.

"Lots of sausage rolls and soft food," Sue said and then whispered in Nina's ear, "probably for all the false teeth there are in here."

Nina giggled.

"Might have been better to serve soup," she said and her mum nudged her and Nina flicked her fingers faster.

"Look at Daisy." Sue nodded at her little granddaughter on the dance floor, jumping and spinning. She had somehow managed to pull the bow off the front of her dress and was throwing it and catching it as she went. Running round and round in circles in the disco lights. Funny how it was acceptable for a three-year-old to be completely hyperactive, but not Nina. "Why don't you go dance with her?"

Nina exhaled. She loved Daisy, she really did. And Freddie. They were both so small that they thought she was normal and this meant she could do whatever she liked when they were together. They didn't care if she jumped or jiggled or doodled or tapped. But sometimes she felt like their unappreciated babysitter. Just because she was the youngest, she had to look after the little ones. Maybe it was just easier for them to keep her out of the way.

"I don't feel like dancing," Nina said. "Where's Josh, maybe he could dance with them?"

They glanced round the room. Josh had arrived with someone called Matilda from his work and was now standing very close to her at the bar in a way that clearly said he didn't want to be interrupted.

"Maybe not then," Nina said.

"Looks like he's otherwise engaged." Sue laughed. "Wonder how long this one will last."

"What about Jess? I mean, they are actually her children," Nina said but immediately realised she'd made a mistake as she could see Jess listening intently to an unknown oldie's stories on the other side of the dance floor. As they watched she put her head back and laughed at whatever she'd heard.

"Jess is socialising, doing the rounds." And there it was in her mother's words. The difference between the first-born wonder that was Jessica, with her soft and floaty name that sounded like a whisper, and the last-born fiasco that was herself, Nina, with a name that had made all the boys in the playground at primary school run around going nee-naw as they pretended to be police cars.

"You should get out there too," Sue suggested, and Nina knew she'd brought it on herself. "Go and say hello to a few people. You don't want them to think you're rude."

Her whole hand was jiggling now, and everything inside her bubbled. She wasn't rude. She was never rude. Or not intentionally.

"What time are we going home?" Nina asked and her mother sighed.

"Later," she said, taking a large glug from a glass of dry white wine. "I'll call us a cab. Now, off you go. I'll see you on the dance floor later."

She pushed Nina lightly in the small of the back and Nina knew there was no escaping. Her mum's eyes were boring into her back as she took a step or two in the direction of the crowd.

"And maybe stop shaking your hand," her mum whispered as she went. Nina clenched her hands into fists and set off, skirting the dance floor as widely as she could so that Daisy didn't spot her.

The smell of Old Spice engulfed her as she got closer to the small groups of family and friends, talking and laughing together.

She made her way through, every now and then getting her cheek pinched by gnarly but well-meaning fingers, or answering the same set questions from a different wrinkly face.

"Ah Nina, how are you?" – "Good thanks."

"How's college?" – "Good thanks."

"How are you enjoying the party?" – "Good thanks."

None of which were true answers, but Nina hope they kept people happy.

Eventually she got to the corner where her grandmother was holding court. She gave her a quick wave and ducked behind to the balloons. To where her pops stood, looking happy but slightly bemused by the whole shenanigans.

"Hi Pops," Nina said. "Happy anniversary."

He put his arms out and she stepped in for a hug. He smelled lightly of soap.

"You look radishing," he said to make her smile.

"It's a good turnout," Nina continued, mentally thanking her mum for the phrase, however annoying she was.

He looked around him in confusion. "The way out?" he asked.

Nina shook her head. "No, Pops. Just saying that you know a lot of people."

"I've had a lot of time to meet them."

"Were you in the army, Pops?" Nina asked suddenly.

"I did my service," he told her, then pointed at a person in the crowd. "With his dad. That's Neddy Banks' son right there, that is."

He looked at the balloons again, frowning.

"What're the numbers for?" he asked.

"The number of years you've been married, Pops," Nina reminded him.

The Everyday and Far Away

He blinked a couple of times. "Married?" He laughed. "Would you believe it? How many years does it say?"

"Fifty-five, Pops."

He nudged her in the ribs. "Time to celery-brate." He grinned and raised his pint to his mouth.

Nina noticed his hand was shaking and it made her sad.

"Where's Sue?" he asked suddenly and Nina pointed her mother out. Sue had succumbed to an Abba track and was shimmying about on the dance floor.

"Where are the others?" He was scanning the dance floor, his chin quivering.

"Jess is there…" Nina pointed at Jessica and Andy, dancing together with Daisy and Freddie holding a hand each, like the perfect happy family they were.

"And Josh is there…" she said and pointed at Josh, who was now kissing the woman from accounts.

"He's obviously hungry," Pops said and she giggled.

"What about you?" he went on. "Have you brought your young man with you?"

She sniffed at the thought of Taylor Jenkins being called a "young man". She didn't think he was as developed as that.

Pops looked laser-sharp at her, eyes bright buttons under his bushy grey eyebrows.

"I heard you had a boyfriend. Nan told me."

She felt something block her throat and shook her head.

Since she'd spent a bit of time with Taylor, she'd gone off the idea of being his girlfriend. All he did on the few occasions they'd met up was throw chips at pigeons in the park and make fart noises as people walked past to laugh at their reactions. She hadn't returned his texts after that and soon her phone was silent again. It had been a relief, to tell the truth.

"I think I liked the idea of him more than I liked him," she said on a sigh. "In fact, I definitely thought more of his motorbike more than I liked him, Pops."

He nodded at something he could empathise with.

"He still hasn't mended that knocking either," she added.

"He'll pay for that down the road," Pops said. "Plenty more fish in the sea, TillyMint."

Nina screwed up her face. "I guess I just jumped at him because he liked me, Pops. Because most people don't, actually, like me at all."

"Why not?" he asked, taking another trembly mouthful of beer.

"Because of all my 'stuff'," she said, shrugging but wanting to cry. Her leg jigged but it didn't help.

"What stuff?" he said and Nina thought maybe he'd just forgotten.

"You know, my attention thing. My concentration."

Pops shook his head. "That's nothing. You'll find the right person. Someone who likes you *with* all your stuff."

Nina bit her lip and he elbowed her very gently in the ribs.

"You will, you know, TillyMint." Pops put his pint down carefully on the round wooden table next to them. "I had these to contend with," he said, pulling his two flappy ears out of the side of his head like Dumbo. "And look who I got." He nodded over at Nan and smiled like he'd won the lottery.

Nina couldn't help but smile back.

"You all right, Ernie?" a fella in a shirt with a button missing over his beer belly called over. "Need another beer?" He motioned drinking with his hand as though Pops was deaf as well as old and Pops gave him a thumbs-up and a wink. The man bundled off towards the bar and Pops sank the rest of his pint in readiness.

"Who's that?" Nina asked, wondering where she'd seen him before.

"No idea," Pops said with a shrug.

The Far Away

1958

Basic training for national service was a shock to the system to say the least. The day we arrived, they shaved my head almost to the crown, leaving only a small mat of hair right on the top. Although everyone else was in the same boat, my ears stayed red all day, embarrassed as they were now really on show. And the language shouted at us made some of the boys' eyes widen. Not so much me, I was a bit more used to Alf after he'd had a few pints on a Saturday night. Usually cursing at his own boots as he stumbled around the bedroom trying to take them off. Sarge yelled so loud that spit sprayed my face and tiny little blood vessels burst behind his eyeballs.

We'd come a long way since we all lined up for our medicals naked as the day we were born. Nurses with straight faces stood either side of the line and stuck you in both your arms with a needle. One boy passed out cold and white on the floor and we had to step over him till he got up again. The nurses didn't bother at all, just bent down to him and jabbed him while he was unconscious. After that it was for the doctor to inspect us, from teeth to backside, and I was glad to get my clothes on again. My new uniform. The scratchiest, most uncomfortable thing I'd ever worn. Two sizes too big on the bottom and pulled in with a belt. My boots as solid as though they'd been set in stone. It was when I had to bundle up my civvies and mark them with my address to be sent home that I first missed Alf. An image of him on his way back from the stall, boiling the kettle for a cuppa, made me press my mouth firm shut.

The next six weeks turned me from a skinny whippet to a wire. The rations were never enough. We scraped our bowls clean and tried to savour any flavour, but my stomach still growled at night in my bunk. We paraded – badly at first until the sarge shouted at us that we looked like a "set of pregnant women on parade". We lined up, tallest to shortest, me somewhere in the middle. We marched. We drilled. We went on exercises. Any scrap of fat I'd had on my body soon fell off. My ribs stood out in ablutions when we stripped to wash.

The boys were friendly enough, though some more than others. We lined up next to each other every day; we slept next to each other at night. I bunked next to Neddy Banks, from the countryside in Devon. I was lucky with him, because he only occasionally snored, but not enough to keep you awake. He grew up on a farm and had big muscles in his arms, from milking cows he said. "Bloody big cows," I said, which he thought was funny.

We spat and polished our boots together on our beds in the evening. The spit on my shoe reminded me of Dot and the hiss of the fire. I told him about her and he told me about his dog he'd left behind on the farm. The one he'd had since a pup who used to sleep on the end of his bed at night. Ned missed putting his feet on something warm in the barracks. The solid security of it. The heartbeat against his soles. Although I'd never had a dog, I knew he was describing the same thing that I felt.

It was a longing for home.

Phyllis crept into my mind often. The tilt of her neck as she showed me the shoes. The widening of her eyes when she saw me in the shop. I played our conversation again and again in my head over the first few weeks, trying to reassure myself she got the hidden message. I was not interested in the shoes. I was talking about her. She had everything I wanted.

I'd only seen Alf once since I left. He came to the presentation at the end of basic training. I wasn't expecting to see him, although I'd told him about it in a letter. He wasn't a writer really, Alf, his letters never said much, just a bit of gossip from the market. Maggie Edwards from the baker's was taking up with Blackie the Sweep. Budgie's parrot had laid an egg. So when I saw him that day right at the back of the crowd – but a head taller than anyone else and easy to spot – a lump stopped me swallowing for a good minute. After we got our final handshakes from the sarge, the sarge then shouted, "Them what's got parents 'ere, get orf to see 'em," and I marched to Alf with a puffed chest and he shook my hand and clapped my shoulder at the same time.

"Look at you, boy," he kept saying. "Would you look at you."

Ned's family couldn't take time off from the milking so Alf pumped his arm up and down too. He took us for a pint and a pie at the pub and laughed his big laugh and was too big for his stool and then I didn't see him again for a long time because we were sent to Cyprus.

I'd been picked out in basic training for the motorbike. Having my licence saw me good and they earmarked me early doors as a despatch rider. I couldn't have been happier than that day, after a four-hour fatigue and rifle training, to be told that when we got to Cyprus I'd be the one running the messages by motorcycle between the units. At that point, anything that gave me a few hours off my feet was welcome. And Cyprus was a ticket everyone wanted, seeing as there was no real fighting by then, just peacekeeping the belt.

Riding a motorbike in the military was a very different matter to riding round Bromley, especially in Cyprus. It wasn't like taking Liberty up the high street or to the pictures. It was hotter than I'd ever known, even more so with a helmet on keeping all your heat in your head. The sweat came right through your uniform and we all stank like dogs as we went into the tents at night. When I removed my helmet and goggles, what was left of my hair lay flat and wet on my head, and my ears fair flapped in relief at having the air around them.

Ned and I shared a tent in Cyprus. We lay next to each other in the dark and listened to the wind blow the tent flaps about in the relief of the heat of the day. We heard the dogs barking and the guards change through the canvas. In the early days, we talked late into the night about the noises we missed. Me, the noise of the birds waking up in the morning as I got up for the market. The sound of the barrows on pavements as the other traders set up their stalls. The sound of Alf whistling as he shaved his whiskers. Ned, the sound of the cows as he walked towards the shed. The cluck of chickens. The clatter of pans in the kitchen as his mum made dinner.

But as time passed, we got more used to it, not just the darkness of the sky, the warmth of the winds, but the sound of each other's breathing, the way we fell into step beside each other on the way to the breakfast tent. It began to feel like we'd always been there. Like I'd known him for ever. Like he was my brother.

The bike I rode was a 350cc Matchless. It was painted green and was faster than Libby. It was rougher in its guts and because of that I called it Ruby after the landlady of the Nag's Head on Fenwick Street who smoked too much. Ruby started reliably and had panniers on the back for me to carry documents and papers to the different units, or to Limassol to the head office. Every day after rations I'd report to the office tent and collect my orders. Every day, I'd ride an hour or so, along patchy roads and into foreign towns. Kids would wave at me from the roadside and I'd beep my horn at them in return. The actual handing over of documents needed a salute and some respect, but then I was back on the bike again, dreaming of the one I'd get when I was home. A Norton Dominator. I'd ride to the shoe shop. I'd been sending my £15 per week back to Alf, religiously. By the time I got back, I was hoping it would be enough, if not immediately, then soon. Phyllis would hear me pull up outside, the throatiness of the engine showing its quality. She'd come out of the shop, smoothing down her apron against her thighs. She'd pause at the kerb and see me there, taking off my helmet. She'd see I was a man of my word. I played the scene through in my head every afternoon, trying to work out the first thing I should say to her. But words were not my strong point, and after six months I still had nothing more than hello.

When the other boys got letters from their sweethearts, I watched their eyes go soft as they read them. I saw the way their mouths moved as they went over each word to take it in. I wondered often if I should have asked Phyllis to write. But it would have been too much, too soon. We didn't know each other well enough to know what to say.

I'd fix that when I got back.

Normally my duties were finished by two, and our afternoons were spent playing football – which I was never good at – or resting, until one day the truck turned up and offered everyone a lift to the beach. We clambered in, and when we got there it was a wide empty strip of sand with the bluest sea. I'd only ever seen the Mersey in Liverpool or the grey-brown waters of the dock and it took my breath away.

Ned was first in, stripping off his clothes, throwing his trousers back over his shoulder and running naked towards the water. We chased him into the waves, we whooped, we hollered, we splashed each other. Nobody could swim but we ran and kicked and sat on the beach until the driver called us back again and we stumbled sandy and sunburnt into our uniforms and onto the truck. I wondered if Alf had ever swum in a sea so warm or Phyllis had ever felt the sand between her toes. I wanted to show them both how it felt.

Just over a year later, I got my demob date and so did Ned. I wrote to Alf and finally let the excitement build in my mind.

Six weeks later, Ned and I buckled up next to each other on the shaky military aircraft back to England. We took one last look at the endless blue skies and the next time our feet hit ground we saw the grey skies and smog of home. We took the same train into London, rattling along towards our homes. And then he clapped me on the back before hugging me tight on the platform before he took another train – a smaller, slower one – out to Devon, back to the farm. I watched it go. For the first couple of weeks, I'd looked for him at my side. If I woke at night I listened for his breath. And I knew that it would never matter how much time went between us seeing each other again, Neddy Banks and I would always be able to sit next to each other, chatty or quiet, and be happy.

Alf met me outside the station. I wasn't expecting to see him, thinking he'd be packing away the stall. But there he was, waving at me across the road, and for the first time ever as I crossed towards him I didn't feel small in comparison. And when we shook hands, I felt like a man.

Over a pint in The Sovereigns straight off the train, Alf asked me question after question about Cyprus and the army and my friends. He asked after Ned, and then I wondered about who would be riding my Matchless now. Whether they'd toot the horn at the kids the same way I had. Alf asked about the temperature of the sea, how many clouds were in the sky. He wanted to know everything. He shouted to the men from the market: "Look who's back, boys," he said, clapping me on the shoulder and making me sway in my chair. They raised their pints at me, they called their greetings, and they put a drink for me behind the bar.

Then, over a second pint I bought, Alf carefully removed an envelope from his trouser pocket and pushed it across the table towards me, careful to avoid the beer puddles around our glasses.

"What's that?" I asked, full of dread.

Last time he'd held an envelope towards me it meant two years away in a hard bed. This time, he just nodded at it, indicating I should pick it up with the faintest hint of a smile. Between my fingers, I realised it wasn't a letter; it was fatter, padded almost. I opened the flap and saw a wad of money, all notes with a few loose coins at the bottom of the envelope. I clutched it shut again, glanced around me to check nobody had seen.

"That's all your pay, that is, Ernie."

"I told you to use some of it," I said. "To keep the flat and to cover my part of the stall."

"Didn't want to do that. And business has been good since they built that new office block at the end of the high street. We've loads of new customers. That's for you to get what you've always wanted."

I could hear my breathing in my own ears. I licked my lips, almost unable to believe my eyes. We both knew what the money would be spent on.

"A Norton Dominator," I said quietly. I opened the envelope again and licked my finger before leafing through, counting as quickly as my wet digit could move through the notes. He was right, there was enough, even though Nortons were more expensive than Triumphs or a BSA. It was the motorbike I'd always wanted. Had my heart set on it for years. Something about the shape, the sound of the engine, it stood way above the rest as far as I was concerned.

"Your own motorbike," Alf said with a wink, and I realised he was proud. Of me and of himself. His chest was pushed out but his eyes were soft. I tucked the envelope safely in my inside pocket, reached over and shook his hand, pumping it up and down over the table until he laughed and shook me off.

Over the third pint, when his words came out easier, he told me everything he hadn't written in letters. The fact that his knee was "giving him gyp – especially on rainy days" and that Estrella had left the market. "Gone off back to Spain to live with her sister." He missed her, he said. Her space had been filled by Nicky Nixon – who was in truth called Arthur but that never stuck – who played piano in the pub for a knees-up. The fact that Alf had won at cards three weeks in a row, and Budgie wanted to do double or quits. Finally, the fact that he and Peggy at the pie shop had struck up a friendship. A special kind of friendship, he called it, and then concentrated fiercely on the bottom of his pint as he took a long pull.

I felt things shifting under my feet, just like when I'd stood in the sand at the sea's edge.

"But I wanted to know what you thought about that," Alf said when he placed the jar back on the wooden table between us. "Before I carry it on."

I raised my eyebrows, not sure what I thought, truth be told.

It was not something I'd been expecting him to say. All the years we'd been together, he'd never been out with women. He'd not whistled anyone on the market the way the other men did. He'd not even looked as Busty Betty walked past, and I'd seen men with their jaws hanging open in her wake. In the early days, when we first left Liverpool, he'd cry about Mam if he had too many beers. Big heaving shoulders and silent tears that frightened me with their weight. I'd stand beside his chair and put my hand on his shoulder, hoping he'd stop and muss my hair, or give me a playful poke in the arm to show he was back to normal. Years later, there were times when I'd still catch him with a faraway look and he'd scrub at his eyes when I came in the room.

But more recently, he'd smile as he remembered those people we both missed. He pointed out something that Dot might have liked or a dress that Mam would have worn well. And every year on their birthdays, he'd buy us a little cake to share and blow out a candle for them. It had become a tradition and he never missed it. Mam's was always pink and Dot's always had a rosebud of icing on it. "Cos she never got much bigger than that," he'd said once.

I'd not thought of him with anyone else. It just hadn't crossed my mind ever. At the beginning I'd worried that if he met someone else he might still give me away. But with each day, month, year that had gone past, I'd realised Alf was sticking with me.

Now, he held my eye even though I could tell he'd rather look away. I noticed the grey in his beard now. The crow's feet by his eyes.

"You know she'd never take your mother's place," he said then, and my heart stopped me saying anything at all.

"A different breed was my Josephine and I'll miss her for ever," Alf continued and my eyes got hot. He shrugged, as though to reassure me. "It's just nice to have the company, what with you being a man yourself now."

I nodded, thinking about what I knew about Peggy from the pie shop. She was a nice woman, always floury up to the elbows. Always hot-looking about her cheeks. Always smiling. I wondered briefly if Alf just liked women who smelled of baking. And then I smiled at the thought of my mammy with the butter bits at the end of the day.

"That's nice," I said at last with a nod. "I like Peggy."

I watched him blow out a big lungful of air as though he'd been holding it. I wondered how long he'd been wanting to tell me and how long it had been a secret in his head. It brought my own secret to mind. Phyllis Marshall.

"I like Phyllis more though," I said. "For myself I mean," I hurried to say when Alf frowned in confusion. "That's something I've been thinking about a lot while I've been away."

I felt the flush of blood in my neck, it being the first time I'd said it out loud to anyone apart from Neddy. And especially to someone who knew her, like Alf. He straightened on his stool, shifted slightly in the seat.

"Didn't know you were still carrying a torch for her."

I thought of all my hours spent thinking of her over the last two years. The time on my bike, when I'd imagined pointing out mountains and beaches to her riding behind me. The quiet times outside the tent when I'd imagine what it would feel like to sit with my arm round her shoulders. The time between waking and sleeping when I'd think about how it would feel to be able to say goodnight to her each evening and good morning the next day. All the hours, the imagined conversations, all based on five minutes in the shoe shop. I took a deep breath and nodded.

"Time to do something about that now," I said and took a long pull of my pint.

Alf fixed me with a look. "Think it's a bit too late to be doing something about that actually, Ernie," he said, and grimaced like his teeth were hurting him.

I met his eye, and I could feel the air in my mouth as I waited for him to say whatever he was going to say.

"Phyllis Marshall's engaged. She's getting married next month."

I got through the next few weeks in a daze. The happiness to be home had been stolen away and replaced by a dull ache where I thought my heart must live.

Alf had tried to buoy me up, when he'd seen my face fall at the pub. He told me everything he knew, as though knowing all the facts might help it to sink in, but I still shook my head every time I thought of her. How could she have not known? How could she have not waited? I didn't understand and I had no way of finding out.

The one thing that made me happy was Josie. My new bike.

She was black and chrome. She was second-hand but only a handful of years old, and she was beautiful.

Alf had come with me to check her over. He watched as I ran my hands over her flat-bottomed petrol tank, her leather seat. I tested the cast-metal brake and clutch levers. I buffed the spotlight on the front. When I looked at him to double-check my instincts, he nodded his approval. She was perfect. I paid for her, counting the notes carefully over the counter, thinking of the years they'd taken to save. Then we'd put our helmets on and Alf had ridden alongside me for the first time ever, both of us feeling the wind buffet our chests and the road under our thighs.

Josie ran like a charm. No flat spots on acceleration. No vibration. I ran her gently to start with and then as we got to the country roads I opened her up and laughed out loud at the sheer joy of riding. I just wished I could take my helmet off and feel the wind in my hair, but a promise was a promise and I'd never ride without. Even if my ears did get pressed flat to my head.

It was only when I parked her up outside the flat and ran my hand over the dual seat that I felt the sadness again that I had no need for a second seat. Not any more.

The day of the wedding arrived, a bright and sunny Saturday and I realised I wanted it that way for Phyllis. If she was going to go and get married to someone else, then at least let her have nice weather and a good day.

Alf kept giving me new errands to run from the stall. Deliveries to make. Supplies to collect. But I knew he was just trying to keep me busy till after noon. Then she'd be someone else's wife and there'd be nothing I could do about it. At eleven fifty exactly he sent me out to get a box of bananas from the wholesalers and told me I could take Josie and make a trip of it. He slapped me on the back and then squeezed my shoulder as I put my helmet on and I shut my mouth firmly together, knowing I couldn't even talk if I wanted to. Better to be off on Josie. Better to be gone.

I saw him shake his head as I pulled away.

I cruised round the high street, wasting time. I turned off towards the docks. I was approximately three miles away at noon, when Phyllis would be standing at the altar.

It was then I saw him. Phyllis's fiancé. Standing on the pavement outside a pub, far away from where he should be. I knew who he was. Alf had told me his name and I remembered him from before I left. George Fellowes. He did the books in an office in town. He'd gone to the local grammar school, so his head was full of the right stuff, but he didn't have the kind of face that looked like it laughed very often. He stood there now, his face as white as flour, swaying slightly in his wedding suit.

I slowed down, pulled to the kerb. Why was he here? Maybe he needed a lift? As I dismounted a few feet away, another man came out beside him, older, with a moustache and a waistcoat.

I took my helmet off, confused. Pretended to fiddle with the front wheel so I could hear, so that I could understand. Neither of them paid me any attention, they were far too caught up in their own dramas.

"You should go and tell her at least," the old man said but George Fellowes shook his head fiercely and put his hands through his sandy hair. It stuck up thinly in points.

"I can't," he said.

The old man checked his wristwatch before grasping at George's arm. "She'll be there waiting now, George," he said.

"She'll get over it," he said, and then, "I can't do it," roughly shaking the other man's hand off him. He closed his mouth firmly, a thin tight line, then turned and walked away. I watched him as he zigzagged up the street, heading vaguely in the wrong direction. Away from the church. Away from Phyllis. Away from married life.

I watched him go. Half of me wanting to run after him, turn him round on his heels, and hurry him to Phyllis so that she wouldn't be humiliated. The other half of me wanted to watch him leave and be sure that he was gone. The older man stood watching him too and, when he saw George turn the corner without looking back, he threw up his hands in frustration and barged back into the pub.

I didn't hesitate. My heart was banging and my stomach hurt for Phyllis. All I could think of was her standing, waiting for someone who wasn't going to turn up for her. The cruelty of leaving her on her own pierced my heart as though someone had done it to me and I threw my leg over Josie and kicked the stand out of the way. I navigated a tight U-turn in the street and roared off back towards St Joan of Arc Catholic Church.

When I pulled up outside ten minutes later, it was clear the wedding party knew the ceremony wasn't going ahead. This was not a delay. It was not someone running late. It was a desertion.

Mrs Marshall sobbed into a white lacy handkerchief next to a fuming Mr Marshall at the church door. A group of guests wandered nearby, smoking and talking quietly, all wide-eyed and nervous, flicking glances around as if hoping George might materialise out of thin air. I left Josie parked on the gravel and took my helmet off as I crunched up the path, still unsure as to what I was going to do. Scanning both sides of the churchyard, I couldn't see Phyllis. A clutch of young men kicked their toes in the stones by the first row of graves. A gaggle of women whispered behind their hands. I walked through their muted conversations, trying to look like I belonged.

"So humiliating."

"Cold feet."

"Never be able to walk down the high street again."

I turned at the last comment, fixed my eyes on the young woman with pencil-thin eyebrows who'd said it, wondering if she was talking about Phyllis or George. My heart hurt thinking Phyllis would be the one that came out worst of this situation. Like she was damaged goods or something.

I edged past the crying mother and into the church. Sunlight streamed through the stained-glass windows. Dust motes sparkled in the air that smelled heavily of incense and antiques.

The priest moved around the altar, busying himself, then coughed discreetly and disappeared behind a curtain to the left. The seats sat empty. The organ was quiet. I paused in the arch of the doorway, then spotted her, sitting alone on the front pew.

Her back was straight but looked as though it would fold if anyone touched her. She held herself so still, so taut, that I could imagine her spine inside, every knuckle of it balanced perfectly on the one beneath, holding her upright, keeping her together.

My boots sounded hollow on the tiled floor. I realised I was holding my breath until I could see her face. I reached her side and she turned to face me. I still had no idea what I was doing there but I couldn't let her hurt on her own.

It was the face of shock rather than the face of devastation. Her cheeks were sucked in by the clasp of her teeth on her lower lip. Her eyes were blank and wide, as though unseeing. When she recognised me, they widened even further, if that was possible. Her hands were clasped round a small posy of flowers tied with string in her lap. Her dress was white and plain with long sleeves. Her hair was pulled up behind her head in a style that made her look older but suited her cheekbones, her skin.

I felt angrier than I'd ever felt. We looked at each other in silence. I cleared my throat.

"Need a lift?"

Her lips parted slightly as though to speak but nothing came out.

"Thought you might want to get out of here."

She took a deep breath in and let it slowly out again and that was enough for her to make a decision. She stood up and I took her elbow, in case she faltered. But she didn't.

She walked out beside me, head held high. The conversations stilled as we passed the congregation. Her mother called after her but she didn't turn.

When we got to Josie, I mounted first and she climbed on behind me, pulled her white skirts out of the way of the wheels. I saw the open mouths of the girls, the frown on her father's face and all I cared about was getting her as far away as possible. Somewhere she could let her spine soften, let her shoulders slump.

Somewhere she could cry.

As we bumped out of the churchyard and she gripped the sides of my jacket between her fingers, I realised she'd left her posy on the pew.

The Everyday

Someone was holding on to my arm. A man. I tried to shake him off but he tightened his grip. He was smiling at me like some kind of grinning ninny. I glared back at him. He rang a doorbell on the door in front of us, still holding my sleeve. The sound was an old-fashioned bing-bong. Reminded me of somewhere.

"Soon have you back," the man said, like a nodding dog.

It was hot and I was itchy and uncomfortable. I twisted my arm away from him, but he was intent on holding on. I growled at him instead.

He looked a bit surprised at that, and rang the bell again, twice.

There was movement behind the glass, and then Phyllis opened it, wiping her hands on a pinny.

"Afternoon Phyllis," the man said, jovially.

Phyllis took in the two of us standing in front of her and rolled her eyes.

"Where was he this time?"

"Down by the market. Looks like he left in a hurry so I thought I'd better bring him back." He pointed at my feet. I looked too. I didn't have any shoes on. Maybe that was why my feet hurt.

"Ah love," Phyllis said to me, "were you off on your adventures?"

She put a hand out to me and I took it. I'd rather hold hers any day of the week than this fella's.

"He loves it down the market," she said, helping me through the doorway, into the cool. "It's his old stomping ground. I hadn't even noticed he'd gone."

"Is that what you were doing. A trip down memory lane?" the man called to me, in a voice that was loud and slow. He turned to Phyllis and coughed in embarrassment. "He actually told me he was off to make a delivery – to you!" He laughed and I bared my teeth at him.

"That's not very nice, Ernie. It was kind of Nigel to bring you home."

Home. There were photos on the wall. Boys, girls. Motorbikes.

"He seems to be wandering a lot, though, Phyllis. What about when the weather turns. What if he wanders off then?"

Phyllis pulled me into the hall and pointed me at a door, then patted my back as I went past.

"Go and have a sit-down, love. You must be tired."

I shuffled towards the door. The carpet felt nice under my feet.

The man was still on the doorstep, watching me. I stuck my fingers up at him as I went into the room just to show him I was still cross. He widened his eyes and took a step backwards.

"Look, I'll leave you to it," he said. "Give us a shout if you need anything, Phyl. I'm only next door."

"Thanks again, Nigel. Bless you."

The chair in front of me had one of those nice footrests in front of it and it fitted me perfectly when I sat down. I groaned out loud, it was so good.

"Honestly Ernie. What were you thinking?" she said as she perched on the footstool by my feet. She inspected them gingerly, holding them each by the big toe. "No harm done," she said. "This time."

Her face relaxed and she reached forward to hold my hand. I gripped it. I felt safe when she held me hand.

"Home now," she said, with a smile that was just for me, and I felt better. Like the sun had come out.

"Where were you off to then?" she said as she shoved my feet into their slippers.

I cleared my throat; it felt like a long time since I'd said anything.

"Was going to stop in on Alf," I said.

She looked at me for a long time, and then kissed me on the forehead.

Nina

Nina and her mum walked to the shop in the mornings, with sandwiches in their bags they'd made the night before. Cheese for Mum. Peanut butter for Nina. A packet of crisps each. They would choose some fruit from the shop for afters.

They wore the same branded t-shirt, the shop's logo on the right chest. **ALF'S**, it said above a shiny red apple. ***The Family Grocers*** it said beneath. Sue had had them made when Pops left the shop to her and decided to take a "back seat". Not that he wasn't always popping in and out.

Less so these days though. Much, much less. Nina wore her black hoodie over the top of her uniform until the last minute, when she had to take it off.

Sue and Nina knew the route would take twelve minutes to walk and they left at eight forty every morning in order to arrive and open up by nine. Truth be told, they'd fallen into a bit of a routine and Nina was stuck in it and spiralling in it, and not sure she'd ever be able to escape.

Her mum was normally already irritated by the time they left the house, tapping the front door key against her leg as she waited for Nina to come out with one shoe still to put on, or without brushing her hair.

"You can't be seen in public like that!" Sue would say. Or, "You do realise you're working with customers, don't you?" Or her personal favourite, "You're the representative of the family brand in the shop, Nina. Smarten yourself up."

The walk to the corner would be brisk and frosty, whatever the weather. Nina always had to stop and call the tortoiseshell cat on the corner and give him a little tickle. She felt like he waited for her and she didn't want to let him down. Her mum would tut quietly or look at her watch until she stood again. Usually Sue had softened a bit by the time they got to the park, when Nina told her about last night's dream or pointed out birds.

This morning, Nina saw the college kids cutting across to the campus. She put her head down and walked faster until they were out of sight, making her mum puff and ask her where the fire was.

Mum talked about *EastEnders* and *Line of Duty*, and how Nan and Pops were. And how bad Pops' memory was getting and how now some of the things he was doing made it dangerous for him to be on his own.

"Like what?"

"He forgot he put the gas hob on. He could have started a fire."

"Wonder what he wanted to cook?" said Nina, thinking about how Pops loved a pie more than anything. Or a fresh pastry, like a cinnamon roll. He used to wink at her before he took the first bite.

"It doesn't matter what he was going to cook, Neen. He could have been making a Black Forest gateau for all I know. It's the fact he forgot about the hob," Sue pointed out.

Nina nodded and shrugged at the same time. To be honest, she'd done that too. Only once. She turned it on to heat water for pasta and then started a puzzle in her bedroom. The pan boiled dry and the smell was awful and then the smoke alarm went off and Sue had made a right fuss and said she wasn't to cook unless she stayed in the kitchen the whole time. Which meant Sue didn't yet realise her youngest daughter didn't have to leave the room to forget what she was doing.

"And last week he went out in the middle of the night and left the front door wide open while Nan was asleep in her bed. Can you imagine?" Sue's voice was very concerned.

"Where did he go?"

"What do you mean where did he go?"

"I was just wondering…" Nina said, thinking if he might have gone round to Alf's old house. He'd done that before. Knocked on the door and everything. The people that lived there now had had a right shock. Or maybe Pops had gone to the allotments. He used to take her there when she was little and let her pick the berries.

"It's not where he was planning on going—"

"I get it," Nina cut in, irritated. "It's the fact he went out."

"Exactly." Sue seemed happy Nina agreed with her. "Just think, he could have gone anywhere, all on his own in the dark and cold. He only had his pyjamas on."

Nina imagined her pops creeping down the road in the dead of night, like a figure in a cartoon. The old man in *Scooby-Doo*, or something like that. She grinned, then saw Mum looking at her out of the corner of her eye and quickly straightened her face.

"When did Nan realise he'd gone?"

"The police picked him up on the high street and brought him home. Luckily he's well known around here. The first thing Nan even knew about his little excursion was when two policemen appeared on her – open – doorstep to bring him back. She was so put out."

Two policemen had once visited Nina at school. Well, not her, individually, but the whole class. They'd told them all about the job and how a career in the force was a great choice. They'd talked about solving mysteries, busting drugs gangs, saving trafficked children. At no point did they mention taking old men home in their pyjamas.

"The doctors and the social are starting to think it's time for him to go into a home." Sue sighed. "But your nan's hanging on in there. She wants to look after him herself, you see. Till death do us part and all that."

Then Sue glanced sideways at Nina. "Talking of love, any other fellas on the scene? Since the wheelie wonder?"

Nina shrugged and kicked a stone along the pavement.

"I know I shouldn't say it, Neen, but I wasn't surprised that didn't work out."

"Why?" snapped Nina. "Because I'm too weird for a boyfriend?"

"What? No! Because he wasn't good enough for you! I mean, wheelies and TikToks and burgers." Sue flapped her hand dismissively.

Nina's mouth dropped open.

"Just because he liked you doesn't mean he was right for you. The right one will be out there somewhere soon." Mum bumped her with her hip as they turned the corner. "And he'll be ON TIME too."

Nina felt something inside. Nerves. Hope. Disbelief. She wasn't sure which.

"Do you really think so?" she asked quietly.

Her mum grabbed her in a side hug and pulled her in. "I know so," she said into her hair.

Nina leaned in, just for a second, against the familiar shape of her mum's body, and thought the feeling might be hope.

"Key," Sue said as they approached the shop door.

Nina had closed up the night before when her mum got a call to go to help Nan put Pops in the bath.

Nina panicked for a split second that she didn't have it, but then put her hand in her pocket and felt it there, smooth and cold. She exhaled to herself, feeling a mixture of pride and relief as she passed it over under the green and white stripe of the greengrocer canopy.

They flicked the lights on and took their aprons from their hanging hook. Sue turned the power on at the till and the radio. Nina started stacking the display boxes in the window space.

Sue opened the back door to access the cold store out the back and bring in the vegetables she kept there overnight for lasting freshness. And then she made a very loud noise.

Nina knew something was wrong. The exclamation was a mixture of shock and dismay. Nina gulped. She knew instinctively that whatever had happened, it would be her fault. And just after she'd thought things might be going right between them.

"Nina!" Mum barked from the back. "What was the last thing I asked you to do last night?"

Nina closed her eyes. The cold store door needed closing and locking as well as the front door. She fluttered her hands beside her thighs and eyed the door, fleetingly considering legging it along the high street rather than see the expression on her mum's face. As if she'd conjured it, her mum's face appeared round the door.

"Come in here," she said and pulled her head back out of sight. Nina dragged her feet to the back door while her insides started to fizz and turn. The cold store was essentially in the backyard. You had to step out of the shop and into the store, just one footstep across the concrete patio. One very important step that separated the shop from the store and meant that it was really an outbuilding.

The cold store door was wide open. Her mum's position blocked Nina's view until she was almost at her shoulder. Then she saw what she'd done. She'd let the mice in.

The boxes of rice were lined up on the top shelf, apart from the one nearest her, which had a big hole gnawed in it and the rice was spilled in tiny pyramids. The box of carrots on the floor had also been attacked. There were several half-chewed carrots on the top. The floor had a scattering of mouse droppings on it. Nina felt her eyes prick with tears and stammered an immediate apology, hating herself. Why had she forgotten to lock the store?

"Look at it!" her mum said, waving her arms. The open boxes of broccoli. The tray of lettuces in their cellophane wrapping. The corn on the cob laid in neat rows. All were potentially contaminated.

"I'm so sorry, Mum," Nina said again, but her mum was shaking her head.

"We'll have to throw it all away. Can't take the risk." Mum put both hands in her hair and Nina wondered if she was going to cry. "A shop in Manchester got fined £4,000, you know, for signs of mice in the shop."

"I remember locking the back door…" Nina said helplessly, trying to make things better.

"Well, thank God for that, otherwise they'd be in there too. So why didn't you do this one at the same time?" Sue demanded. "Look at the waste, Nina! Look at the cost."

"I just forgot…" Nina said, remembering the music she was listening to on her headphones as she locked up, 'New Rules' by Dua Lipa, as she thought about how she wanted to make up her own rules and not have to go back to college and study anything to do with retail. She didn't want to have to run a greengrocers when she was older. And how very much she wanted to break out, be free, find her own way.

She'd turned the music up loud. She'd actually felt the tiniest glimmer of excitement about her imagined future. She'd make some friends. She'd meet another boy, one that she actually liked this time. She'd sung out loud as she put out the bin. She'd even danced a bit as she mopped the floor in the shop.

Then she'd locked the back door, put the mop in the cupboard, hung up her apron and left. Taking great care to lock the front door, and check it was locked three times before going home.

But she left the mice to have a very big party.

"Honestly, it's one thing after another with you, Nina. When am I going to be able to trust you to be left on your own? When am I going to not have to worry about every little thing?"

That stung.

Nina opened her mouth to say something but her mother wasn't finished.

"I just long for a day to myself, and peace and quiet. A whole day. Just one. The luxury! I'd go and have a massage or get my nails done like other women."

Nina couldn't help but glance at her mum's hands with her nails short and unpainted, with normally a bit of dirt still there from the veggie displays. Wrinkled and rough.

"But you never get your nails done," she pointed out.

"Exactly," Sue said meaningfully and Nina realised this sounded like an accusation. As though it were all Nina's fault. Everything.

"I don't know who I'm supposed to be more worried about," Sue finished in a tired voice. "You or Pops."

Nina ran out of the shop and raced home to bounce on the trampoline for a very long time.

The Far Away

1960

Daily deliveries to Phyllis became the norm after she got jilted. After I dropped her off that strange Saturday, and she clambered stiffly off Josie, she whispered only one thing before opening the door beside the shop that led up to the flat where she and her family lived.

"Thank you."

The door closed quietly between us and I imagined her slumping against it the other side. Leaning on it for support, as she cried.

I watched the blue paintwork for a couple of seconds in case it reopened but it was impenetrable, shut.

By the time I got back to the market, without the supplies Alf had sent me off for in the first place, the news had spread.

Phyllis was back home unwed and George had run away.

The gossips were at work already as to what she'd done, why George Fellowes had chosen to leave his place of birth rather than marry her. The market was full of it.

Alf just asked how she was. Phyllis.

I shrugged.

"Silly question, I s'pose," he agreed.

Later when he heard what I'd seen, George deserting her, he understood why I'd gone. Why I couldn't leave her there alone.

"She'll need a bit of time," he said the next day.

"She'll also need a bit of care," I added, lifting a small punnet of the ripest strawberries from the stall. "Don't worry, Alf, I'll pay for them." He waved a hand at me in refusal and off I went. The shoe shop was closed. It was Sunday and everything on the high street was quiet and blank. My knocking on the blue door to the flat echoed on the pavement.

Her mother opened the door that first day.

"She doesn't want to see anyone," she said, sniffing, but I saw the way she wrung her hands together, and wondered who else had been round. Or whether in fact nobody had called at all. I imagined Phyllis listening to see who it was. Had her heart started beating fast in case it was George?

"I'm Ernie," I said, loudly enough to travel.

"I know," the mother said and something about that gave me hope.

"I brought her some strawberries." I held the punnet out and she looked at them as though she'd never seen strawberries before. "From the market." But she still didn't take them.

"I thought they might cheer her up," I said, pushing the box closer until finally she put a hand out to take them.

"Thank you." She hugged the small box close. "That's kind of you." Then she flicked her eyes left and right to see if anyone else was there before she shut the door.

She didn't expect to see me the next day, this time with some raspberries. Or the next with bananas. Or the one after that with a couple of shiny red apples.

She stopped looking surprised after a week. She started greeting me by name after a fortnight. She started looking interested in my offering by the end of the month, almost as though excited by it.

The Everyday and Far Away

Every day I'd sneak a look past her in the doorway to see if I could catch a glimpse of Phyllis, but the hallway was always empty. Once I thought I heard her sneeze. Once a dog barked.

I'd delivered every different type of fruit on the stall three times before I parcelled up the cherries. And it was that day that Phyllis opened the door herself.

It was August by the time she smiled at me for the first time, and this was when I told her I'd found a mouse sleeping in the potatoes on the stall. It was September the first time she let out that tinkling laugh of hers with the story of Budgie losing a bet and having to run through the market in his underpants. October when she agreed to a walk in the park and we sat on a bench together on a damp, foggy afternoon, in public. In November she came to the pictures and we sat in the dark, me not able to concentrate on the film at all as her elbow touched mine on the armrest between us. In December I kissed her goodnight on her father's doorstep and it was better than all my dreaming in Cyprus.

And in May 1961 I got down on one knee in Bromley Park and asked her to be my wife. She took my hand and said yes.

Everything was perfect. I couldn't believe I'd won her heart, and I would do anything to keep it. The one thing that stood between us was Josie.

After her one trip on the bike after being jilted, Phyllis had made it quite clear she didn't want to climb on Josie again.

"I'm not really a motorbike kind of girl," she said with a little lift of her shoulders, apologetic almost. I told her that was fine – everyone to their own – and I kept my riding solo, pulling up outside her door and parking Josie there until I rode her home again later.

Phyllis and I would walk to the park. We got the bus to the pictures. Occasionally her father gave us a lift somewhere in the back of his motorcar.

For a while I persuaded myself it was just a matter of time. I could change her mind. I believed I could get her to like it if she'd just give it a go, but she was adamant.

"It's not ladylike," she insisted, with a toss of her hair.

And that was that. Because I wanted her to feel ladylike. I wanted my dear Phyllis to be happy, always.

As the wedding approached, she started to make noises about us getting a car. The first time she suggested "selling the bike and using the money" I had such a stab of pain in my chest that I thought it might be a heart attack. Once I got my breath back, I could see Phyl's reasoning.

We wanted to travel places together. It would be more practical, she said.

But I couldn't imagine letting go of Josie. Not ever. She was too important.

We'd spend all day together when the market and the shop were shut, walking, sitting in the park if the weather was fine and then an afternoon tea, or a pint for me at the pub.

"What is it you don't like about her?" I asked on one of our Sunday walks, as though Josie were a person and not a bike.

Pulling the sides of her coat in tight against the weather, Phyllis shrugged. "I think it's the straddling. I feel a bit like I'm riding a horse." She gave a self-conscious laugh.

The word "straddling" did funny things to my innards, in the region below my belt, and I shook my head to clear the thoughts.

I *had* to find a solution to keep Phyllis happy but still keep Josie. And I had now just a couple of months to do it.

It came to me in a flash one day on the stall. It was a simple solution, a compromise that, although it hurt me to think about, might solve the problem.

I told Alf what I was thinking. He blew his cheeks out in surprise, and then shook his head. "You must really love her."

"I do."

"Well then," he said. "Let's get it sorted."

A visit to the bike shop, a trip to a mechanic and it was done.

Alf shook his head again as we left, this time in pity.

A week later, Phyllis and I stood together in church in front of Alf and her parents and a gaggle of market friends and shopkeepers from the high street.

She wore a different white dress and her hair was tied in a bun at the back of her neck. We held hands throughout the short service and I felt my ears get hot when I said my vows. But I meant them, every word.

And I listened to her voice, clear and confident, as she repeated them back to me.

"For better for worse. For richer for poorer. In sickness and in health. To love and to cherish. Till death us do part."

When we walked out of the church, pink-cheeked, beaming, excited and terrified that we were married, the moment of truth was here.

Josie was parked just outside the churchyard. A bow of white ribbon was tied to her handlebars. Attached to her side was a low-level, seated sidecar for Phyllis. It had a covered front so that she could be dry and warm, and a small visor to keep the wind off her face.

Alf had told me it would change the way I rode, but if it meant we rode together then I felt it would be worth it.

I turned to see her reaction, heart in my mouth for the second tine that day (the first was when waiting for her to walk down the aisle, thinking about how she'd felt the first time). But then she'd appeared in the church doorway and the organ had played and Alf gave me a wink from the front row, and I knew I'd never been happier.

Now, I stood waiting.

Phyllis stopped still and stared. Then she clapped her hands in delight and kissed me full on the mouth. "Ernie!" she said into my smile. "You're a good man."

"Thank you cherry much," I said back and she broke into laughter.

This time we took her posy with us. It sat in her lap in the sidecar, as we pulled away laughing and waving and beeping the horn.

It was the start of the sidecar days.

The Everyday

Phyllis is quiet lately.

She's got that worried look about her. The same one as when she watches something on the telly to do with hospitals, or policemen. Like she's got a weight on her shoulders and a crease between her eyebrows.

Every time I put my hand out to her, she still squeezes it in hers, but it doesn't make her smile. It seems to make her sad.

I caught her watching me in the bedroom. I can't remember what I was doing in there but she came in and made me jump.

"What are you doing making such a mess?" Her voice was cross, and puzzled.

I looked at her.

And then I saw there were old photos all around me. A box with the lid off. Square black and whites on the carpet, some sepia photos with fuzzy faces. A few brightly coloured ones. Children with no teeth. They all looked happy, whoever they were.

"Be careful with them," Phyllis said after a while and a bit more kindly, kneeling down beside me with a creak, and I tried to grin at her.

Then she started putting them back in the box, stopping to smile at one every now and then, until the carpet was clear.

She took the one last snap that was still in my hands; a girl – hair in bunches, holding a bucket at the beach. Phyllis took it from my fingers and slipped it under the lid and closed it firmly.

She made me biscuits today to go with my cuppa. Cookies she called them but I know what they are. She said it was a special treat and we could eat them in the sitting room. They tasted like treacle.

Sitting next to me, she patted my arm as I nibbled and sipped. She didn't stop me or slap at my hand when I reached for another.

"Ernie, it's time to face facts," she said and her voice sounded like she hadn't slept for a week.

The treacly bits were stuck in my false teeth and I sucked at them loudly, making her jump. I smiled and took another bite.

There was a bird on the feeding table outside the window. Small, fast. Maybe a tit? I nodded at it to show her but she was talking.

"I can't look after you properly on my own any more," she said.

Not sure what she meant, I took another biscuit and this time she caught my hand.

"Are you listening, love?"

I blinked. The bird had a shrill trill and a flash of yellow on its front. Definitely a tit. I nodded again. The bird's friends arrived, attracted by its noise. Maybe he was shouting about the food. They took turns on the feeder, chipping into the peanuts with their tiny, pointed beaks.

"The truth of it is that now you need more help than I can give you." Her voice seemed to catch, and it felt as if I heard it from a long way away.

Phyllis wasn't looking at the birds. She was damp-eyed, dabbing at her face with a cloth, which she then tucked up her sleeve.

I hated seeing her upset and I reached for her hand on the armrest between us as she continued to talk.

But I wasn't listening as now the birds were busy flitting between the feeder and our tree, and I remembered that this feeder was the one that dropped nuts everywhere in the autumn. The little things would take cover under the leaves of a branch before flying back again to get some more food.

Phyllis held my hand to her cheek.

"Everyone says it's really nice."

It *was* nice. Her cheek felt powdery soft against my knuckles and she pressed her face to my hand so hard I could feel her bones underneath. Indeed my hand left a mark when she let it go. I noticed that she'd got more wrinkles than before. When did she start looking like that, so much older than me?

"They'll bring you your dinner on a tray."

The tits were growing in numbers. Three more of them now. Their legs no thicker than a… What was it? The thing you light your fag with. What was it *called*?

"Match!" I cried at last.

Phyllis seemed taken aback but then she nodded quickly.

"Of course you'll be able to watch the match, Ernie. I bet they have a big TV in the lounge," she told me.

On, off. Tree, table. Back for a peanut. Busy. Busy. A bigger bird came down with beady eyes, and scared the smaller birds away.

"Frightened," I said.

Phyllis dabbed at her eyes again.

"Nothing to be frightened of," she said after a while. "I'll come and see you every day."

She put her arms round me then and I had to look over her shoulder to still see the birds. I was glad when the black one flew off down the garden and, a few seconds later, the tits came back. A whole family of them this time.

I smiled at Phyllis as she let me go.

"Ah, Ernie love," she said, pushing the last biscuit towards me. "You're a good man."

Nina

Nina knew Nan needed help packing the house up if she was going to move into theirs now that Pops had gone into the home, but she had a sneaking suspicion that the "new routine" Mum had implemented had more to do with Nina's mistake with the cold store than anything else.

These days, every afternoon at about 3p.m., Sue would tell her to walk to her nan's for the last few hours of the day to help Nan get a 'head start' on the packing. Her mum would then "sort the shop out" at the end of the day and join Nina there later. Nina had apologised what felt like a million times, and had also offered to lock up a couple of times since, but Sue always had a good reason she herself should do it that day.

But Nina knew the real reason. She wasn't considered responsible. Or mature. It was clear that as far as Sue was concerned Nina was considered a loser.

Nina kicked stones all the way to her nan's house and even the cat on the corner knew to stay out of the way.

"Hi Nan," she shouted as she opened the back door, and followed the muffled reply into the back bedroom where she saw Nan on her knees in front of an open cupboard, an empty cardboard box beside her.

"Would you look at this, love!" she said, turning to Nina with a pair of baby bootees in her hands. They were made of leather and had lambswool inners. Real works of art. No

Nike trainers for Nan's babies by the looks of it. Not way back when.

"Such workmanship!" Nan said, pressing them into Nina's hands to admire. They were pink, or had been once, although now they were dusty and faded with age. Nina turned them gently in her fingers, conscious that she was clumsy and might damage them. She could tell they were precious and she would do anything not to hurt Nan.

"Those were your mum's," Nan said, reaching back into the cupboard. "And these were your Uncle Stephen's." She cupped a tiny blue pair in her hands and then pressed them to her own heart, then shook herself and laughed.

"This is why it's taking me so long to sort anything out! I keep starting on one thing and then get distracted!"

"Welcome to my world, Nan," said Nina, sitting down on the carpet beside her.

"So many memories, Neen," Nan said. "A whole life in this house. Babies. Work. Family. Friends. Just think, you've got all this to look forward to!"

Nina sighed. Not at this rate. Stuck in a dead-end job where she wasn't even trusted to lock a door. Signed up to a college course she didn't even want to do.

Nina rubbed the carpet under her palm, this way, that way, making patterns in the pile.

"Are you sad to leave this house, Nan?" she asked.

"Yes and no, really," her nan said. "It's been a good home for me. But it's not the same without your pops in it."

"Have you seen him today?" Nina wrote her name on the carpet with her finger.

"Of course. Every morning at ten thirty, in time for the tea round so we can have a cuppa together."

"How was he?" Nina asked, drawing a sun with beams coming out all around it.

"Not great today," Nan said, her voice little more than a whisper. "He was very angry with me for not visiting. I told him I was there yesterday but he must have forgotten."

"I'm going in tomorrow," Nina said. "And I went in Sunday. I'll try to cheer him up." She wiped away her pattern with one big stroke and the pile looked perfect again. If only everything was so easy.

"I know. You're a good girl." Nan patted her hand and then gently she took the bootees from Nina and put them back in the cupboard.

"I thought we were meant to be taking things out of the cupboard, Nan?" Nina said.

"I'm putting things back in the cupboard – for now – that I want to keep safe. I'm just throwing the rubbish away first," Nan said, pulling out an old pile of fabric that looked like it had seen better days. She flicked through it.

Some of the patterns were so 1970s and so buoyant that the oranges and yellows and browns made Nina's eyes go funny.

Thankfully, after a moment of consideration, Nan dumped the whole bundle in the cardboard box.

"What shall I do today, Nan?" Nina asked. Over the last week, she'd cleaned out kitchen cabinets, and taken the plates and bowls to the local hostel. She'd put all the spare bedding and sheets in the community recycling bin. She'd emptied out a display cabinet of video tapes. None of which could be played any more as nobody she knew had a video player. They had writing on them saying what had been recorded, and then it was crossed out and the new programme written underneath. Nan obviously used to like to watch *Dallas* and *Knots Landing*. Pops liked westerns, whatever they were. Nina also took a whole box of old CDs to the market and sold them to the new bric-a-brac stallie for £10, which her nan let her keep.

"Could you do Grandad's wardrobe, love?" Nan said and passed Nina a box. "I can't face it. It can probably all go to Cancer Research on the high street. He's got everything he needs at the home now, and everything should have been washed or clean before it went back in the wardrobe. Box it up and Mum can take it in the car when you go."

Nan turned back to her cupboard and Nina went into their bedroom, which looked the same as always, apart from only the one set of pillows on the bed. Still on Nan's side, though. That hadn't changed.

Otherwise, the wooden ducks still flew up the wall, the family photos still smiled at the bed, the vase of plastic flowers still sat on the windowsill.

Nina stuck her earphones in to help her concentrate – well, as much as was possible.

As she opened the wardrobe doors she got a waft of the smell of Pops. Warm, clean washing. Wool and cotton mixed together. She sniffed it in and thought of him at the home. He'd been pleased to see her the other day. He called her by name. He whistled a bird song. She'd grabbed a puzzle from the games table in the corner and arranged it on the table between them. It was their thing and it gave them something to do while she was there.

He'd rubbed his hands together in glee, but never put one piece together all the time she was there. She got stuck in, piece by piece by piece, until the old-fashioned photographic shot of a stream and a meadow was put together. When she looked up at him with a smile, she realised he'd nodded off. He seemed to sleep a lot these days.

Now, she emptied his wardrobe quickly, throwing things randomly to the floor, but then choosing the right garment to fit in the next spot in the box, by shape, by size, by texture. Could she roll it? Should it lie flat? Was it bulky? Treating the job like a puzzle was the only way to get it done. She tried not to look at the individual pieces as she packed them.

Then somehow she had three full boxes and Pops' shelves were empty. She looked around and decided that across the house the bulk of the sorting and the packing up was done, and that her own mother had managed to avoid quite a lot of this hard work. But Nina didn't mind as she liked to be active, and helpful, and Nan had certainly needed her help. And she felt Nan appreciated her efforts, which was nice.

Nina was about to shut the doors when she spotted a lone item at the back of the top shelf. Reaching up, she hooked it with her fingertips and pulled it towards her. A single black leather motorcycle glove. She stuck her hand inside it to try it on but hit resistance. A crinkle. A noise. She reached her fingers inside and tweezed out the obstacle. A letter, sealed in a white envelope. On the front, in a black shaky biro, it said,

TOP SECRET

Underneath it said,

FOR PHYLLIS

And underneath that, it said,

FOR WHEN I DIE IN CASE I FORGET

Nina felt the fizzing rising up and she started jogging on the spot.

She could hear her nan humming to herself in the other room, oblivious. She held the letter up to the window, flapped it backwards and forwards in case she could read anything through the paper. A flash of guilt kicked in and she had to spin round in a circle a few times till she felt better.

Unsure as to what to do, she took it back to the spare room, where her nan still had her head in the same cupboard. It was getting to the point that Nan had to make decisions about what she wanted to keep and what she wanted to throw, and the only person who could make that decision was her.

"How you getting on?" Nina asked when Nan's head appeared.

"I don't think I can take any more today." Nan looked little and old and very, very sad. "Everything is so hard. This is our whole life here in this house."

Phyllis looked about her, made a sweeping movement with her hand as though showing Nina everything at once. Her lips were pressed tightly together as if to keep everything inside. Nina knew that feeling.

"Time for a cuppa," Nina said, making up her mind in an instant that Nan did NOT need a top-secret letter today. And didn't it say "For when I die" on its front anyway? She'd save it. Pops was nowhere near dying, was he? Surely someone would let her know if that was the case? She had plenty of time to decide what best to do with it.

The Everyday and Far Away

Nina stuffed the letter in the front pocket of her hoodie and helped Nan to her feet as she creaked upright and then stretched.

"Ernie's motorbike glove," Nan said quietly, taking it in her hands as they went through to the kitchen. "That man loved that bike, Nina, he said it made him happy all his life. It's out there in the garage, you know, gathering dust."

Nan flicked the kettle on and lifted two china mugs from the mug stand, then sat down heavily in a chair, obviously tired.

An idea struck Nina. One that would help Nan out and might give her some Brownie points with Mum as well. A job she could do on her own to show she *was* responsible and she *could* be trusted.

"Why don't I concentrate on the garage now then, Nan?" she suggested. "There's not a lot more I can do to help in the house. I think it looks like we're at the point where you need to make the decisions as to what stays and what goes."

Nan wiped her hands on her thighs, a motion that took Nina back to the shop as a little girl when her nan would dust her hands off and give her a strawberry.

"I haven't been out there for years, it was Pops' domain," Nan said, considering the garage idea. "But I do know that the only thing worth keeping out there is Josie. Everything else could just be cleared out."

The kettle flicked itself off and Nina poured hot water on the tea bags in Nan's old mugs.

"Maybe if there are any tools you could sell them to the market?" Nan said.

Nina got the milk from the fridge and topped up their drinks.

"I could start today!" Nina felt a buzz of excitement that she might actually be doing something right.

"Let's leave those teas to cool off a bit, and we'll go and have a look, love," Nan said, pulling her cardigan around herself and opening the back door.

The garage was at the bottom of the back garden, opening up onto the back lane like all the other garages on the road did. Many years ago Nan had got Pops to fix a trellis up it and now a rambling rose covered most of the side facing the house. Nina heard Nan tut as she walked towards it, and mutter that the rose bush needed pruning before the house went on the market.

"One more job to add to the list," she sighed as they reached the end of the path. She twisted a few thorny branches away from the door before she put her hand on the knob and turned, but nothing happened. She tried again, grunting with effort.

"Is it stuck?" Nina said, having a go herself but with no more effect than her nan. They both stepped back to look.

"No," Phyllis said, pointing at the rusty keyhole. "It's locked."

She blew out noisily, and Nina felt her plan falling apart.

"And Ernie would have had the key," Nan said. "So, heaven knows where that is."

She turned away, shaking her head, giving up on the idea already. "Come on Neen, our tea will be getting cold."

The Far Away

1963

I wanted a shop and Phyllis wanted a baby. It wasn't that it was a "one or the other" kind of situation, one took hard work and money and the other took luck, but we spent the first two years of our married life trying for both of them.

We had the choice as newlyweds of moving in with the Marshalls in the flat above the shoe shop, or living with Alf in his flat above the bookies while we saved up money for our own home. I was surprised when she chose Alf's. Not because I wouldn't – I would, every day of the week – but because I thought she might want to be in her own family home.

"No way." She laughed. "Much easier to be the woman of the house if my mother's not about."

So that's what she became. The woman of our house. Alf was happy with the arrangement he said, and so after our wedding weekend in Dorset we moved back in as man and wife.

Phyllis knocked our rooms into a proper home. She added a tablecloth and armchair covers. We suddenly had a tea served up to us every night at the same time when she got back from the shop, rather than a pie left over at Peggy's or a bag of chips. She shooed Alf's feet off the sofa and sometimes there were even flowers on the windowsill that you could see from the high street outside.

We settled into living together. I got used to being her husband and Phyllis got used to being my wife. I liked to hear her humming to herself in the kitchen. The way she put her arm through mine as we walked home from work, or would huff a proud little breath on her wedding ring and then buff it on her sleeve to keep it shiny.

She said I made her laugh. Even when I wasn't trying. It would tinkle through the house like a bell. She was the first thing I saw in the mornings, waking early to watch me as I pulled on my braces ready for setting up the stall. She was the last thing I saw at night. "See you in the morning," she always said.

"If you're lucky," I'd say back and hear her smile in the dark.

We saved like mad. Every week we made the trip to the bank together and put in everything we could. Alf had always taught me to save a third, spend a third, live on a third. But for those two years we spent hardly anything and saved half our wages every Friday. We didn't need a lot of money for entertainment anyway. "Baby-making's free," Phyllis used to say, whispering the words in my ear so that nobody else could hear. "Thank God for that," I replied. "I'd be broke." She nudged me and pretended to be outraged but I knew she was pleased really.

Our only luxury was the fuel for Josie and our Sunday outings. We'd pack a sandwich lunch and tuck it by Phyl's feet in the sidecar. Then we'd be off, riding somewhere new each week. Sometimes to the countryside, the Surrey Hills maybe, through big green forests and past wide-open fields. Other times we'd take to the coast, the Lanes of Brighton. Canvey Island, land on one side of us and water on the other as we rode along. We'd find somewhere nice to park up and sometimes take a little walk, and decide on somewhere to sit, eat our picnic and share a flask of tea looking at a new view. That's when we'd make our plans and admit our dreams to each other. That's when I told her I wanted a shop. The stall was taking its toll, the early visit to the wholesaler, the setting up, the pulling down. The temporariness of it. The way Alf's hips creaked as he went up the stairs to the flat made me see he needed somewhere he could sit behind a counter in a few years. I wanted a greengrocers for our future. I saw us all in a shop.

Phyl talked about babies, us having a little family of our own. She told me she wanted more than one – if we were blessed that way – saying she'd never liked being an only child, and I had to agree with her on that score. She looked shy as she suggested middle names for the children, Dorothy if we were lucky enough to have a girl. That made me well up and I pretended the wind was in my eye.

The dreams started coming true of their own accord. The shop first came to us unexpectedly. Phyl's father and mother invited us for our tea on a Saturday night. It was even quieter in their house than normal, as they were never ones for the wireless or music, so often the hiss of the fire was the only noise in the sitting room. That night they sat on the edge of the settee and announced they were moving to Clacton. It wasn't a total surprise, Mr Marshall had been talking about retiring for a few months, but we hadn't imagined it to be so soon. We thought he'd stay another few years at least. But an opportunity had come up for them to move nearer to Mrs Marshall's sister and they wanted to take it.

"We're not getting any younger," said Mrs Marshall, and I thought how much older they seemed than Alf with his whistles and winks. But in fact, they were probably a very similar age. "But we want to see the two of you set up before we go."

Mr Marshall cleared his throat and outlined the plan. We could buy the shop from them and move into the flat above it. I held my hand out to stop him as I felt the colour start in my collar, knowing the shop and the flat together were way out of our sights price-wise.

But then he named a figure, and I had to ask him to repeat it. It was more than reasonable. It was fantastic!

Phyllis clutched my hand in hope, and I felt my brain straining to work out what we had already and what we'd need. With a few quick calculations of our savings, I decided we could do it.

We'd need a mortgage but the savings we had were more than enough for a deposit and I told myself the bank wouldn't turn us down.

Phyllis and I shared a look, both of us knowing this was the move we were looking for, before I turned back to Mr Marshall and extended my hand.

"Thank you, Mr Marshall," I said, as we shook hands. "It's a deal."

"I think it's about time you called me Ted," he said just as Phyllis hugged her mother.

June 1964 the first delivery of fruit and veg arrived and in the closed shop I showed Phyllis how to make a pyramid with the apples, how to lay the potatoes in straw. She herself added little touches of her own, red ribbon on baskets, chequered tablecloths under the jars of jam. It was a far cry from the buckets of potatoes on the stall.

We'd bought a weighing scale and the stainless-steel bowl shone like silver, she'd polished it that many times. There was a till at the counter and a stool behind. We added some tins on a shelf behind the counter, selling a few odd and sods, as well as sweets and tea.

But the main display was the best fruit and vegetables we could find. We organised them in baskets and trays and punnets, vegetables one side of the aisle, fruit the other.

The window display had the deal of the day. Buy three, get one free. Or a special price promotion. Three for a sixpence, that kind of thing. I'd come up with the promotion and Phyl wrote it on the slates so that anyone passing by could see we were good value. Then when they came in, they could see we had a good range and we only sold quality produce.

Alf had been telling everyone for weeks about our grand opening while we worked at removing the shoe shelves and installing what we needed after the stall was packed up for the night. For weeks the shop still smelled of leather but now it smelled of earth and apples and fruit skins and fresh air.

"What it's to be called?" Alf said, many a time. "The customers need to know."

"Not sure yet," I said, teasing.

"Ernie's?" he said, nudging me. "Ernest's? Or just The Greengrocers?"

"It hasn't come to me yet." I gave a big shrug.

It had come to me though. I was just waiting for the sign to be painted.

On opening morning, a small crowd were gathered on the pavement. Phyllis, Alf and I stood in our aprons, beaming. Peggy from the pie shop was there; Budgie and some of the traders had traipsed up, leaving others to mind their stalls. A gaggle of young mothers stood with their baskets and shopping bags ready. And I noticed Annie from The Sovereigns there, and she asked if I might be able to set up a supply for the pub kitchen. And I was thrilled as, if I could get her on board, the other pubs would follow.

Never a one for words, I thanked everyone for coming and said they all got a free bag of apples to take home with them.

And then I pulled the cloth off the sign to unveil it and there it was in big bold black writing. **ALF AND SON**.

And underneath, **A FAMILY BUSINESS**.

Alf's mouth fell open as he looked at it. Everyone cheered and then they started filing past me into the shop. I could hear the young women exclaiming about the cabbages, as big as my head. The carrots, tied together by their frilly green tops.

"Is it all right?" I asked Alf, who was still staring at the sign, as suddenly I felt awkward that I'd called myself his son. In writing. In public. And without asking him first.

Alf shook his head as if he couldn't believe his eyes.

"It's more than all right," he said as he threw an arm round my shoulder.

I noticed he wasn't quite as tall as he used to be, or maybe it was that he wasn't quite so upright. He slapped my back, one, two, three times before looking at me.

He wiped the corner of his eyes and shook his head again. "I'm the proudest I've ever been, son. The proudest I've ever been."

And now it was my turn to feel overcome with emotion.

Later that day, when the floor had been swept, the till tallied and the three aprons hung up next to each other on hooks, Alf went off whistling to pick Peggy up so they could go for a pint. I turned the hanging sign in the window to "closed" and looked out into the dusk of the high street, watching all the other shopkeepers going through their own closing-up routines. The hardware man in his overalls dragging his boxes in. The baker wiping down the shelves. The butcher closing up the cold stores. I admired my new view of the shops opposite. The slate of the rooftops. The sound of boots away up the pavement. I finally felt like it was real. Our new home.

Phyllis came up behind me and put her arms round my middle. I held her hands against me at the front. I could feel her chin jutting into my back as she rested her head there.

"Where have you 'bean' all my life?" I asked her and felt her laugh.

"It was a good first day," I added. "Met lots of new customers and Annie's going to give us a trial for the pub."

The wind picked up outside and a couple scurried past, chins tucked into their coat collars.

"The sign went down well too," she said and I glanced at it out there, swinging silently on its well-oiled hinges. She repeated the wording. "A family business."

I heard her take a breath, a big one, and then let it out.

"It's perfect, Ernie, because our family's going to be growing in a few months."

I twisted to look at her over my shoulder but couldn't see her face. I swivelled in her hug and held her away from me, just so that I could see.

A nervous, excited flush was on her cheeks as she let go of me and pressed both hands to her tummy.

I whooped. I kissed her. She laughed and I kissed her again.

"You do know what this means though, don't you, Ernie?" she said, grinning.

"Of course I do, you daft thing," I said. "You're having a baby!"

She rolled her eyes and shook her head.

"Yes. We are."

I hugged her tight, happier than I'd ever been.

And she said, quietly in my ear, "Which means we're going to need to get a car."

The Everyday

We were all sat in chairs angled towards the big screen in the room with a window to the garden, although they always put me facing the window rather than the TV, knowing I liked to watch the birds rather than whatever was showing on the television. It was mainly rubbish. Big wheels being spun. People pressing buzzers. Sometimes jumping up and down on the spot. I didn't know what all the fuss was about. But the birds were making their nests outside and I loved to watch. The little ones with straw. The bigger ones with twigs.

My stomach growled and I craned my neck to see out of the door towards the room where we ate our dinner. I could smell something cooking, so it couldn't be long till lunch.

"What's for lunch?" I called to Marina, one of the young girls who helped us with our meals, as she walked past. I remembered her name and I'd told her they used to make a car called a Marina. She'd smiled at that and said she'd never seen one. She couldn't be much older than my Susan.

"You've had your lunch, Ernie," she said with a laugh and I frowned. "Chicken pie. You cleared your plate."

Chicken pie? I like chicken pie. My mouth watered again and she patted my shoulder before moving away. Was she going to get me a pie?

A woman came in the main doorway, wide-hipped, big-bosomed, talking to one of the people from here. The uniform ones. They were laughing together. They saw me looking and both waved. I waved back politely and they both grinned. Some of the people here were all right really.

I liked some of the old ones, like Cyril who always shouted too loud because he was deaf himself. And Marjorie who liked to sing in the afternoons. You could hear her down the corridor, trilling away like a canary on Budgie's stall. They were cheerful enough. But I liked Gerald the most. He used to have a Triumph. Rode it all the way to Cornwall and back for a holiday.

I avoided the narky ones. The woman who stabbed any elbows rested on the breakfast table with her fork, telling people it was bad manners. Brian who only spoke to tell you to shut up because he couldn't hear the telly.

Some of the young ones were nice too. The black girl with the plaits on her head who helped me with my walking, holding my hand like she was sweet on me. She never minded if I was slow. The boy with the crew cut that made him look like he'd just come out of the army who would always give me an extra sugar in my tea. He used to tap the side of his nose like it was our little secret.

I didn't like the grey-haired woman down the corridor though. She sat behind a desk and would stop me at the door whenever I wanted to go out and look at the birds.

"You know you're not to go out there on your own, Ernie," she was always saying like I was some kind of child. She'd lead me back into the lounge, where she'd plop me into a chair I didn't want to sit in, one where I couldn't even see the garden. I waited a few times until she was away from her desk and got to the door as quickly as my gammy old feet would carry me and tried the door, but she'd always locked it. One day I'd get past her, I'd promised myself.

All I wanted to do was go in the garden. What was the harm in that?

Phyllis had asked them to hang a bird feeder right outside the window and she brought nuts from the stall when it needed filling. The birds loved them. We had blue tits and sparrows the most. Occasional wood pigeons that just strutted around under the feeder to eat the fallen seeds. But the best ones were the goldfinches. They arrived in a little flash of yellow, so tiny and beautiful.

I'd always tell the person in the next chair if they made an appearance. Unless it was Brian. I didn't bother telling him. He'd just tell me to shut up and shout at someone to turn the effing telly up. The first time he swore at me, I told him to watch his language, what with Phyllis being next to me in the chair. But it made him worse and he started effing and jeffing, and Phyllis nudged me and put her finger to her lips, trying not to laugh, and we both shook silently as we looked out the window.

I like it best when Phyllis is with me. She sits with me and we hold hands between the chairs. It makes me feel better. She comes some days and not others but she always insists she comes every day and so I let her think I believe her. She comes on the bus, she says. I don't know why she can't just come and stay here too. I've asked her a few times. And sometimes I ask her whether I can go home with her. And then I'll ask again whether she can stop with me. But she can't, she says. She has to go. I know she doesn't like me asking either as it makes her face go funny. But I can't help myself.

The wide-hipped woman was making her way around the room, talking to everyone in their chairs. She knew everyone apparently. Even the mad ones I kept away from. Some were nasty, some were mean. She was holding hands, or crouching down in front of people to talk.

"Nice to see you," she said to one of the old girls who'd forgotten to put her teeth in.

"How you doing today, Doris? Feet okay?" to another lady with her feet up on a stool.

"Maurice? Have you done the crossword yet?" to the man who always had a newspaper on his lap but never spoke as far as I was aware. There was a wave at one chair, a pause at the next. She was coming my way.

I glanced out the window again just in time to see a bird on the feeder, upside down like an arrow.

"Nuthatch," I said to Betty in the chair beside me and pointed outside. She peered at it though her glasses, made a little noise and turned back to the TV where someone was looking round a big house. Couldn't she see how clever the nuthatch was, balancing upside down to eat? I snorted.

"Look, Ernie, who's here to see you!" the woman with plaits said and there she was in front of me with the wide-hipped woman, who was holding out a chocolate bar. My favourite. A minty Aero. Her eyes were the bluest blue. They reminded me of Phyllis.

She smiled a big soft smile and I couldn't help but smile back. She was so happy to see me. It felt nice that smile. Like standing in sunlight on the stall.

"A-ha!" I said, rubbing my hands together, excited to see the chocolate and feeling good in the smile. Betty looked at me, to see what was going on. I indicated the woman in front of me and puffed up my chest. "Here she is! My girlfriend."

The woman gave a little chuckle and handed the chocolate over. "Ah, Dad. How you doing today? Seen any goldfinches?"

She gave me a kiss on the cheek and moved a spare chair next to me, and we watched out the window together for a while, sucking chocolate and watching the birds.

Nina

Nina had the letter hidden in her sock drawer. She looked at it at least once a day, but normally probably a dozen times. She'd held it to the light again, peering for clues. She'd picked at the seal, just a little bit, with her short, bitten fingernail, half-willing it to open and half-wanting it to stay shut. She traced the writing with her finger, knowing it was her pops', even though it was Nan who always wrote the birthday and Christmas cards. She'd seen his script on the calendar at their house, and on boxes in the garage. A long time ago, on the fruit and vegetable labels at the shop. She knew it was his writing, his letter, his secret.

That word raced through her every time she read it, making her fingers tingle until she clapped them together or shook them out. After she put the letter back in her drawer and covered it up, she always got really wired and would have to put her music on loud so that she could dance it out for a little while, or until Mum shouted up the stairs or banged on the door.

It had been a week since Nina found the letter and since then she'd helped Nan every day and worked in the shop too, where she had tried to stop annoying people by being too jumpy, or jiggly, or just there. Mum had softened, but still insisted on locking up the shop herself, so that it felt to Nina that nothing was changing. It made her frightened that this would be the routine for the rest of her life.

The only place she felt she didn't get on people's nerves was at the home on Wednesdays and Sundays when she visited Pops.

The Everyday and Far Away

He was in the main sitting room when she got there. Everyone else was watching the TV so loudly it made her wince, but Pops was staring out the window instead.

Nina picked her way through the chairs all arranged in the same direction, careful of old legs in nylon trousers and slippered feet that stuck out all over the place, and she found a footstool to perch on by his side.

"Hi Pops," she said, leaning in towards him.

He turned to look at her, but his eyes were unsure. They didn't light up, and instead stayed flat and questioning. A surge of anxiety flooded through her. This looked like one of his bad days. She'd heard Nan and Mum talking about when he seemed lost in faraway days. When he didn't seem to be in the everyday at all.

"It's me, Nina. Your TillyMint."

He looked out the window again and pointed a gnarly old finger at the bushes. A blackbird. They watched it hop across the lawn to the borders where it disappeared into a bush. A few seconds later, it emerged with a worm in its beak and Pops turned to her with a big grin.

"That's a big one," Nina said and he whistled, which made him dribble slightly on one side of his mouth.

"How are you Pops? You okay today?" Nina knew not to expect an answer, but she was ready to be surprised at any time. There seemed these days to be no rhyme nor reason as to when or if he spoke. The doctors said he was forgetting his language, his words. But every now and then, he remembered enough to answer something or even express his feelings.

"Weather's a bit better today," she carried on, nodding towards the drizzle outside. "A good day for the allotment."

He turned back to the garden and she saw the dribble was starting to run towards his chin. She fished a hanky out of her hoodie and dabbed at it, even though the thought of what she was doing made her feel a bit weird.

He glanced at her to see what she was doing, but he didn't seem bothered by her tending to him.

It was getting harder to visit him and stay for more than half an hour. He didn't even attempt a jigsaw puzzle with her any more. He didn't really talk. Nina wasn't even sure if he knew who she was. By the time she'd had a milky lukewarm cup of tea with him, her chat had dried up and her leg would start jigging and her fingers would start drumming, and soon she'd have to make her excuses to leave before it felt like her head would blow off.

"Off to meet some friends," she'd say, or "Must dash, places to go." Both of which were big fat fibs but made her feel less guilty about leaving him there, sitting in his chair. She already felt the urge to go building inside her and she'd only been there five minutes. Nina mentally kicked herself. She had to make this time with him count. Suddenly she had an idea. She pulled her footstool closer so that nobody else could hear.

"I found your letter, Pops," she whispered. He raised a bushy white eyebrow as though waiting. She bit her lip, not sure whether he was taking it in.

"It was in your motorcycle glove!"

He put his hands out in front of him slowly, as though taking the handlebars of a bike. He revved slightly with his right hand. It was the kind of thing a kid would do.

"Yes, that's right, Pops. Your motorbike," she said, encouragingly. "Do you remember your letter, Pops? It says it's a secret."

His hands dropped to his legs again and he nodded.

Did he understand her? Nina wasn't sure.

"I haven't opened it, Pops. It says not to give it to Nan until you die."

Something inside her clenched at saying these words out loud. It didn't feel right.

His eyes were vague-looking, milky, but they were staring into hers. Slowly, he lifted a bent old finger and pointed at her.

"Me?"

He nodded and excitement bolted through her.

"You want me to look after it for you?" she asked with something inside her that felt like amazement.

He nodded again and dribble welled in the same corner of his mouth, although this time she dabbed without thinking.

"You trust me with it? To do the right thing?"

He smiled, and Nina's chest banged with pride. She had never, ever felt so believed in.

She kissed his cheek, and realised he smelled different. Not the same washing powder, probably.

He whistled and pointed at the garden. It had stopped drizzling but the trees were rustling in the wind. He pointed again.

"You want to go outside, Pops?" Nina asked. At that point in time, she would do anything for him. He trusted her. He smiled a shaky kind of smile.

"Yes," he said gruffly.

She stood quickly, a rush of energy making her want to run round the garden fifty times. Or run home and bounce, as high and as fast as she could.

"I'll get you a coat from your room," she said, and slalomed across the lounge to the stairs. His room on the top floor had a good view across the treetops. She'd found him in there more and more recently, gazing out the window. He didn't seem to want to take part in the armchair fitness or craft sessions downstairs. She took a minute to look at the photographs on the wall, hung there by Nan. Every member of the family had a picture, in a frame. Hers was awful. She looked like a right idiot. She must have been talking when the picture was taken as it caught her slightly open-mouthed, wide-eyed, like she was just about to burst into song. Or laughter. Jess looked perfect in hers. Smooth hair, make-up, nice smile. No toothy grin for her. Nina blew a raspberry at the picture. Not even that could bring her down today.

She found his padded warm overcoat in the cupboard and pulled it out. Before she pushed it shut she grabbed an old raincoat of his for herself. Who cared what she looked like – it would keep her warm while she helped him shuffle around the garden.

It took longer than she thought to get him to the bench outside. It had been hard to shove his arms into the coat armholes, and then do the buttons up. It had taken even longer to take his slippers off and replace them with outdoor shoes that thankfully had Velcro straps.

When they finally got there, it was slightly damp on the wood so Nina made sure he was sitting on his coat, and she pulled his hat onto his head so that his ears were inside, before she settled beside him. She thought for a moment that he probably did all those things for her when she was little and now here she was, keeping him warm, helping him dress, making sure he was steady while he walked. But he trusted her. He'd said so. It was the least she could do.

The blackbird made a reappearance a few minutes later and Nina heard a small noise of pleasure in her grandad's throat, which made her smile. She pulled his raincoat around herself, figuring they could sit for five more minutes without him getting too cold and then she'd take him back in. She plunged her chilly hands into the pocket of the mac, on the off-chance he might have stashed one of his mints there. Instead, her fingers found something cold and small and she pulled it out.

And there, in her hand was a key. With a tag on it that, in Pops' capital-letter handwriting, said **GARAGE**.

The Far Away

1965

Even though I hated driving a car, it was soon full.

Stephen Alfred Edward Dawes came first. 14 January 1965. With ears nice and flat to his head.

He was too small for such a big name to start with, but Phyllis said he had long feet so he'd grow into it. I wasn't sure you could gamble on the size of people in the same way you judged how big a dog would get by his paws, but I was no expert so I took her word for it. The first time I held him, on the hospital ward, my heart got so big in my chest I thought I'd cry.

I hadn't expected the impact of the baby on the house. Even though he was a quiet little thing. A contented feeder. He slept through fairly early. But he turned our house upside down overnight.

The smell of nappies soaking in a bucket in the corner. The feel of his sticky little fingers as he clapped them on my face or mouth. The sound of him breathing in his cot in the corner or of him suckling at Phyl's breast in the night-time.

Customers queued up to look at him in the shop in his pram. Budgie shook my hand till it felt like my shoulder was popping out when we asked him to be his godfather, having already won bets on Stephen's sex and the date on which he might be born, and he thought he was a lucky omen. He brought a cage round that night with two goldfinches in it, as a present for his "young charm", and after that the flat was always full of their chirps and scratches.

The christening was a bright day in May. The ceremony wasn't for me that day, it was for Phyl, and she carried our Stephen around in a white dress looking as happy as she had on our wedding day. I wasn't bothered so much in the God department. Nor was Alf judging by the way I saw him sneak a look at his wristwatch as the vicar poured water on Stephen's head up at the font.

We weighed him every week in the shop scales and sometimes the market would have a bet on that too. There he'd be, lying in a clean nappy as a gaggle of the gambling men would crane their necks through the doorway to see how much weight he'd gained. I knew Budgie pestered Phyl regularly, asking what she was feeding him lately, or whether he'd got a taste for something new, trying to get the inside track. Whenever he did win, he'd nudge me with his pointed elbow.

"What did I tell you, Ernie?" he'd say, nodding at the baby. "He's good luck, he is."

I felt the same. Business was good. Phyllis recovered quickly. She was back in the shop the next week, and her apron did up just like it always used to. The pram would be parked in the back room if Stephen were sleeping and pulled up to the till if he was awake. After a few months he sat in his pram and we'd wheel it outside the shop door in fine weather and leave him parked there in the sunshine. Everyone had a word for him as they came in. Everyone had a smile or a pinch of his cheeks. Soon enough he was crawling and then we had to put a gate across the door to the back room so he could roam about in there without getting under customers' feet as they filled their baskets.

All of a sudden he was toddling about. Reaching up for a hand to hold on to, not caring whether it was me, Phyl or Alf. And he was talking, and waving and laughing and running and it felt like he wasn't such a baby. And then Phyllis told me we had another on the way.

Susan Dorothy Anne Dawes came six months later, just after Stephen turned three. With tiny ears like a mouse, a shock of brown hair that stood up on end and a cry that would peel your eyeballs. The noise that came out of that little scrap of a thing scared the finches in their cage. But her hands would clutch at me from just a few weeks, and even before that she held my heart in her fingers. She had the widest blue eyes that felt like they were looking right inside me, as though she could see something there that I'd forgotten. And she was right, because as she got bigger and held my hand I remembered the feel of sweet Dottie's hand, and I held on tighter.

Phyllis talked about trying for another one a few years later. But I was happy with the four of us. It was a good number, I said, and "kept things nice and even". She'd tried to convince me, but I said I didn't want to chance fate that the next one would have big ears, not with the two perfect ones we had already.

So, night-times, we counted our blessings, checking in their rooms and seeing their flushed cheeks, watching them dream before pulling the doors to quietly and padding along to our own bed.

The urge was still there to ride Josie, but it was hard to find the time. Every time there was a bright day, a light wind, I'd get that urge in the pit of my belly to pull on my helmet and kick the stand free. To explore roads I'd never ridden so that I could get to know them though their bumps, their curves.

Josie was parked in the garage out the back when we moved into our house on Green Street. We needed the extra space when Susie came along and it suited Alf, who sold his place and moved into the flat above the shop, with Peggy the Pie, who was by then a permanent feature.

I polished Josie every Sunday and would take her for a short ride if I could manage it, but it was tricky. I couldn't take off for hours – the days of us packing a picnic for a ride were long gone – and I felt guilty leaving Phyl with the two little ones. They were hard work, clambering and crawling in opposite directions. I realised I needed a reason to ride. Or a bloody good excuse was how Alf put it.

So the Bromley Bike Club was born.

Not that I knew it at the time.

I put a poster in the window of the shop, making the most of the free advertising, and Annie let me put one up in The Sovs too, seeing as I told her our first meet would take place on her premises.

I turned up on the first Sunday of the month, with Alf, fully expecting for us to be the only two and that we'd enjoy a ride together and have a pint afterwards, and then we'd go home.

We parked up outside The Sovereigns and sat on our bikes, saying we'd give it half an hour in case anyone couldn't get there spot on. But three others turned up, a few minutes apart. Peter James puttered slowly down the high street on a Triumph, obviously not knowing where The Sovereigns was. Mattie Black rode in on a BSA, and Mike Norton – who we agreed had the best name for a bike enthusiast – on a Royal Enfield.

After twenty minutes or so of discussing each other's bikes, we adjusted goggles and helmets and set off. I'd planned a route that would take an hour and take in as many sights and use as many good riding roads as possible. We thrummed along in single file at first, me leading the line, Alf behind me. We kept the bikes in check until we were clear of the trafficked roads and then we opened them up on empty long straights. We moved to two abreast and swapped positions, let each other take the lead, passing each other with a dip of the helmet, a mark of respect or acknowledgement, letting the other rider enjoy the full force of their own bike.

When Josie and I were up front, nothing ahead of us but open road, I felt every bit as free and excited and happy as I had the first time I rode her. I felt too the familiar press of my ears against the sides of my helmet but it didn't stop my smile behind the visor. Alf pulled up beside me with a glance and a nod as he had a thousand times before. And I imagined a future ride, with Stephen on our other side, the three of us owning the road together.

The rules and regulations were written down by Mike Norton on a notepad that Annie passed over the bar. There weren't many.

1. The Bromley Bike Club was an independent club for motorbike riders.
2. Owners of any type of motorbike could join.
3. We'd meet every first Sunday of the month at The Sovereigns.
4. We'd organise a ride-out every month, leaving The Sovereigns at ten o'clock.
5. The club was not liable for any accidents on these ride-outs. All members were to be responsible for their own safety and the maintenance of their bikes.

Mattie raised a toast to the "inaugural" meeting as he called it, and we all supped our pints.

Then Alf said we needed a chairman, or president, and that it should be me. I stammered out an embarrassed decline but they nodded and raised their pints again and that was that.

I was the chairman of the newly formed Bromley Bike Club and this gave me licence – and reason – and a bloody good excuse to ride once a month from then on.

Word spread.

I kept a poster in the shop window. Mike ran a fish and chip shop and did the same. Mattie still lived with his parents but he put the word out amongst his friends.

The following month there were eight of us, and twelve the next one and within a year we had more than twenty-five. People joined from further afield because there was nothing like it nearby to them.

Big bikes, throaty ones, British models and foreign imports all roared into Bromley on the first Sunday of every month. They lined the pavement from The Sovereigns on the corner right down the high street. It came to be that the first hour of each meeting was spent walking up and down the pavement and admiring all those wonderful machines.

People who didn't even own motorbikes started coming down for a look, and Phyllis and the other wives started bringing the kids down to watch us ride out together.

I overheard Phyllis telling one of the other women she was "married to the chairman" and my chest pumped with pride.

Some of the other women there had a face like a robber's dog but my Phyllis was beautiful; kind, honest and beautiful.

As more and more spectators started to turn up to get a look at the bikes and watch us leave in convoy, Peggy soon caught on and served an early cuppa and a bacon sandwich from the pub to anyone that wanted it, at a small profit of course.

Stephen ran bike to bike on little legs, finding a new favourite every week. Reaching up for the handlebars of a silver Triumph or marvelling at his face in the reflection of a black BMW. The riders all knew him and let him sit on the saddles, try the various models out for size, attempting to convince him that theirs was the best and the one that he should choose when he was old enough to join us.

His feet didn't reach the footrests, and he clamped his skinny thighs to the sides of the seat, but I saw the look on his face was the same as mine had been the first time I sat on Liberty.

And I could see him in my rear-view mirror as we pulled out, when he'd wave until we'd turned the corner.

"He'll be out with us before we know it," Alf said one time and I prayed a little prayer to someone I didn't believe in to keep Alf with me long enough to see it. Not that he was ill, but he was knocking on.

At the beginning of the meets, Susie was a just a babe in arms, not big enough to toddle. Phyllis carried her about on her hip and Sue pointed chubby wet fingers at the bikes and the bikers she wanted to inspect closer. She always knew what she wanted, did our Susie, even at that age. She was passed biker to biker, smeared visors with baby kisses, dribbled down leather jackets and pulled at moustaches and beards. The men didn't mind. They seemed to like the children being about. Susie was balanced on saddles, swung over handlebars, and one time I saw Gerry Morgan tuck her in to sit in his panniers, Susie clapping her hands in delight and all the bikers laughing around her.

"That's one way to take her with us," Gerry laughed over at me.

Stephen was eight when he started asking if he could come with me to Bike Club. Or the BBC as we liked to call it by then.

Josie was parked on the front lawn. It was a Sunday and the shop was shut and we were getting ready for the Bromley Carnival the next weekend. The BBC had been asked to lead the procession through the town, and it would be a slow ride along the high street in front of the floats and lorries, leading the way to the local park for a picnic.

It was as Stephen was helping me to tie red, white and blue ribbons to Josie's handlebars that he first brought it up. "How old were you, Dad, when you first rode the motorbike with Grandad?"

His little fingers struggled to tie a bow and I put a finger in the middle to secure it in place for him to make the loops. That one done, he reached for another. He knew the story, I was sure, that Alf and I rode from Liverpool to London, me holding tight on the back.

"I must have been ten by then," I said. "The journey was so long that my legs trembled for hours after I got off."

"Why?" This was Stephen all over. One question after another. He wanted to know everything about everything.

"It's the vibration of the road. You can feel everything on a bike, every bump, every rise. It's not like sitting in a car," I told him.

Phyllis leaned back on her heels, taking a break from the gardening in the nearby border.

"I'd much rather sit in a car," she said, stretching her back. "Much more comfortable."

Stephen caught my eye and we made a face at each other, taking care that Phyl didn't see this.

"It's not about your bottom, Mum," Stephen said. "It's about the ride."

He looked at me for confirmation and I nodded, thinking I couldn't have put it better myself.

"There's me thinking you used to love our sidecar days!" I said, and Phyllis flapped a gardening glove in my direction.

"You know I did really," she said. "You and Josie changed my world."

She held me with a quick glance; nothing that Stephen would notice, and I remembered the feel of her climbing on for the first time, manoeuvring her wedding dress out of the wheels.

She turned away to plant some red flowers and I got back to polishing the steelwork, huffing and buffing with my yellow cloth.

"When can I get a bike then, Dad?" Stephen asked, tying another ribbon. They hung like hair from the handlebars on both sides now.

"When you're seventeen," I said, "and then you have to do your test."

We talked about the test, him asking how long it would take, how far he'd have to ride. Whether the man who tested him would drive along beside him to see what he was doing, or whether he'd want to ride on the back. That made me laugh. The thought of the tester on the back with a clipboard.

"What job will you get to earn your money to buy the bike?" I asked, and that stopped him in his tracks while he chewed a lip and thought.

"I'll be a boxer," he said, putting his fists together in front of his face, like the poster outside the cinema for *Rocky*.

"Oh no, you won't," said Phyllis without looking up.

"I'll be a policeman then."

"So you can help people?" I asked. "And catch the baddies?"

"Because I can ride a motorbike," Stephen said as if I was dim, and I laughed again. In lots of ways, he was like Phyllis. He had the same long straight back, the slight gap between his two front teeth. They laughed at the same things, at exactly the same moment as though they shared one sense of humour. But he shared my love of bikes, that was the one thing we had that pulled us tight.

Susie was different. She was more like me. She was more solid, more thoughtful. She put her head on one side to hear the birds, she whistled to the finches in the cage to see if they'd reply. Now I watched her cycling down the close with her friends. Streamers attached to the handlebars of her bike, just like mine. Her legs going like little pistons to keep up with the other older children. She'd never be left behind, kept with the others by sheer determination alone.

Josie was gleaming. She looked as good as the day I'd bought her. The sidecar attachment – and then removal – hadn't done any lasting damage and it had been worth every penny.

Stephen put his hand on the saddle and took a breath.

"Can I ride on the back with you, Dad?" he asked, "for the carnival?"

The Everyday and Far Away

The word "yes" was almost out of my mouth when Phyllis said very firmly, "No."

We both turned to look at her.

"Don't you look at me like that," she said, dusting her dirty gloved hands together and shaking her head.

"But Mum—" Stephen began, but she raised an eyebrow and he stopped talking.

"It would be very slow, Phyl, and he'd wear a helmet," I tried, to see if there was any give. "We're only doing a slow parade and then a little turn round the park."

She stood and I knew that if she put her hands on her hips then there was no talking about it.

Phyllis peeled her gloves off and put her hands on her hips. "It's too dangerous," she said, lips pursed firmly together.

Stephen stood up a little straighter and I had to admire his bravery as he asked, "How old do I have to be then, Mum? To go on the back?"

Phyllis looked at me in surprise as though I'd put him up to it, and I shrugged in return, as anxious to hear the answer as he was.

"Well, you need to be a bit bigger to fit on properly," she said, giving herself a bit of time to work out her response.

Stephen stretched himself up even taller beside me. I didn't want to look in case he was on his tiptoes and I drew attention to it.

"I'd say when you're ten," she said decisively and I felt a glimmer of pleasure. Not that long really. It was a good age.

"Same age you were, Dad!" Stephen was beaming at the thought.

I grinned back. It would be something to look forward to.

"And you're never, NEVER, to ride without a helmet." Phyllis wagged a finger at him.

"I'd never do that," Stephen said, shocked. "Dad always wears his."

"Exactly, and he has to fit his ears in his too," she said, although not unkindly. "So, it just shows, it's always better to be uncomfortable and safe than dead."

She went inside to put the kettle on.

When he was sure she'd gone, Stephen put his thumb up at me and I grinned back. Ten wasn't that far away.

Except Stephen died.

Aged nine and a half.

The Everyday

We were outside, sitting on the bench. It wasn't our garden but it was big enough for a tree and a bird feeder and the sun felt nice on my face. Phyllis had come and put my coat on, and stuck my feet into shoes and here we were. She told me it would be lunchtime soon and that I was having jacket potato. She wasn't eating, she said. She held my hand between us on the seat and we watched the birds together.

"Blackbird," I grunted, pointing with my free hand.

"Right as always, Ernie," she said. "You and your birds. You got to know your birds well, getting up early all those years for the stall."

She turned to me.

"You remember your stall, do you, love?"

"Course."

Silly woman. Not that I said that bit out loud.

"That's where I first saw you. Standing there at the weekends with Alf."

I shut my eyes in the sunshine, letting it turn my eyelids yellow. Sometimes the sun had been hot enough to burn my ears bright red on the stall. Other times the snow had turned my fingers blue. Along with Alf's nose.

"I loved you then from my head to-mat-toes," I said, my voice bursting out of nowhere, and she laughed out loud.

It made me feel good inside.

"What about the shop?" Phyllis said then. "Alf and Son as it was then?"

It was enough to jog my memory.

"Coconuts," I said, puffing my chest out.

Phyllis looked surprised. "Yes, the first shop in Bromley to stock them." She squeezed my hand on the wooden slats between us. "And melons. Can you remember Mrs Gates when she asked how to cook it?" She burst into her tinkle of laughter and the blackbird flew away.

I watched it as it landed in a nearby tree, checking for safety.

"And Budgie came in every day cos he missed you being next to him on the market," she added.

Budgie. I thought of the sight of him running up the high street in his underpants.

"They were good days, weren't they, Ernie?"

I heard her sigh.

I shut my eyes again to rest. The market was as fresh in my head as ever. The corner to The Sovereigns. The sound of pigeons and pushbikes. Calling and cobbles. Men swearing, laughing, grunting with the effort of unpacking. Boot Blakey's metal heel protectors loud on the pavements. The smell of pies in the oven already at Peggy's. The swing of the pub door at the end of the day as the stallies all went in for a pint.

Budgie once told me he wished he had a family like mine over one of those beers. He'd said it would be nice to have someone to go home to. Some little ones of his own. And that he was very happy to have Stephen as his godson, just in case he never got any of his own. I'd clinked my jar with him, wishing him a bit of what we had. A family of his own.

Phyllis was still talking.

"Where's the children?" I asked, opening my eyes.

She blinked, then nodded.

"Susan's at the shop," she said. "She came in to see you yesterday, remember? Said she brought you a bar of mint Aero."

I felt myself frown.

"Remember?" Phyllis asked with a nudge.

I didn't. But I wished I did.

"And she's coming again on Friday when she can get a minute. Because I'll be later this Friday because I've got to go to the dentist." She sniffed, thinking. "That's a thought. I probably need to find out whether you get to see the dentist in here. You're probably due a check-up."

"Stephen?" I asked. The boy. My boy. The one with the freckles. Knees bigger than his thighs.

Her face went strange.

I waited. But there was a bad feeling in me. I pulled at her hand, tugged it to get an answer.

She opened her mouth a little as though to speak and then shut it again.

"Stephen?" I said again. It sounded like I was shouting.

"He can't come, can he, love?"

"Stephen," I said, and I could hear how my voice was different, worried.

"Oh Ernie. Please." Phyllis sounded like she was begging.

"I want Stephen." My heart was banging in my chest like it was trying to get out.

Phyllis pressed her eyes shut for a moment and then when she opened them they were black and bottomless.

"He's gone, love. Remember?"

Gone where?

I shook my head.

Was he in the service? Or had he gone to Australia or was it New Zealand where they sent some kids to live? I was scared suddenly, unsure.

I looked around, but he wasn't there. Had I lost him? I started to move my feet together, to get up, to go and find him, but my legs wouldn't stand up on their own. I banged my hands down on the bench either side of me.

Phyllis jumped and tears ran slowly down her cheeks. "He died, love. It was a long time ago. But he died."

A big dark feeling came up inside me. Like I couldn't breathe and might die myself.

"Stephen!" I called.

Then I could hear someone crying, and I tasted snot.

"Can you help me?" Phyllis's cry was anxious. "Gladys? Over here, please. I had to tell him again. Can you help me get him back to his room?"

Nina

Nan looked like she could hardly believe it when Nina showed her the key.

She stood in her empty lounge, in her almost-empty house where she'd been giving it a last "once-over", and she took off her rubber gloves.

"In his raincoat pocket?" she Nan, turning it over in her hands. "Who'd have thought to look there?"

Nina's heart raced until her nan passed the key and tag back to her. She'd looked after it carefully since she found it, checking it almost hourly in her bedroom drawer, next to the letter, until she got to Nan's again.

"All those hours he used to spend out there with Josie," Nan said, her voice fond as she remembered. "Taking her apart, cleaning her up, putting her back together again. Years ago now, though. He slowly stopped. I probably should have noticed earlier. It must have been to do with his memory." She shook her head. "Who knows how long that key's been in his pocket!"

Nina rubbed it between her thumb and finger as though it might bring her luck.

"So can I do the garage, Nan?"

"That'd be great, love," Nan said. "Save me the job."

Nina's mouth suddenly felt too big for her face and she knew she was doing one of her goofy grins but she couldn't help it. She flicked the key around her finger on its little ring.

"You all right about tomorrow?" she asked her nan, who was moving in with them in the morning. This was the last night she would spend in the home she'd lived in for fifty-odd years. Nina couldn't imagine that. She'd lived in three houses already. Phyllis paused and pressed her mouth together before nodding.

"It's the right time, I suppose, to leave. More to the point, Neen, are you all right about tomorrow?"

"What do you mean?" Nina turned the key as fast as she could.

"Do you mind your old nan coming to live with you?" Nan was watching her very carefully and Nina knew she was serious. The key was a whir on her finger. "I promise not to cramp your style."

Nina snorted.

"I haven't got any style to cramp, Nan," she said and they both laughed and when they stopped, Nina added, "Course I don't mind, Nan. It will be nice, you being there."

Because it felt like Nan really needed it to be serious, just for a minute.

Nan took a deep breath and blew it out.

"The For Sale sign goes up tomorrow," she said. "But I'm sure we can get the estate agent to tell anyone interested that the garage is still to be cleared out."

Nina stopped spinning the key and started throwing it hand to hand.

"I'd like to keep Josie for a while. Mum said we could keep her in your garage. I can't think of getting rid of her yet. Although she might not run so well. She'll have been under a dust sheet for years."

Nina was throwing now as though the key was hot. It barely touched her hand before she tossed it to the other one. Mum would have told her to stop by now. But Mum wasn't here.

"Josie's the only thing of value out there though, love. So you can donate or sell anything else. He's got shelf-loads of rubbish probably. Scrap it if you have to."

"I'll tell Mum I still need to come in the afternoons to sort it out," Nina said. "Then I can do a couple of hours a day. It won't take long." She could already feel the excitement of it. The Josie Project. She'd show her mum she could be trusted.

She hummed quietly, the first line of "We Are the Champions" by Queen.

"Let's go see," Nan said, pulling her coat from the banister and shrugging it on. Nina hummed the song louder, excited. As they made their way up the garden path, Nan tutted again about the rose bush.

"Did you know you can eat roses?" Nina said.

"Really, dear?" Nan said as she let Nina pass with the key.

It was stiff but after a wiggle it turned quietly in the lock and made a satisfying click.

"Ta-da," Nina said as she pushed open the door.

"Light switch is on the right," Nan said, behind her.

Nina reached in and found it with her fingers.

Click.

The overhead strip-light whirred and flashed, and then illuminated the garage with bright, white light. Something scurried in a corner.

Nina stopped in her tracks, taking it in. Nan bumped into her back and then peered round her shoulder to see.

There wasn't a clear patch of floor showing. The workbench was also hidden under a huge mound of unidentifiable "stuff".

And there was certainly not a motorbike there, resting under a dust sheet. The sheet itself hung on a hook on the wall.

The bike itself was in bits. About a thousand of them.

Josie's component parts covered the entire garage. A saddle on the table. A loop of chain on the floor. Wheels, cylinders, fuel tank, and things that Nina didn't even know the names of were all separated, scattered, strewn on the floor.

All the tools to maintain the motorbike lay forgotten. Nuts, bolts, screws, spanners. Wrenches, tools of all shapes and sizes lay around. Some shone dully. Some looked rusted and old. Rags with oil on them, brushes, tins of grease and leather cleaner left with lids off, neglected. A torch lay with a battery beside it. A radio lay on its side. Chargers. Hoses. Pliers. A screwdriver set. Those were just the things that Nina knew what they were. Other items lay piled in the corners, where the scuttling noise had come from.

"Oh dear," Nan said, over her shoulder. "Looks like the last time Pops took her apart, he forgot how to put her back together."

The Far Away

1974

The house was so quiet after Stephen died. The only sound at first was Phyllis weeping.

And then she was so worn out with weeping that she stopped making a noise even though the tears kept rolling down her cheeks. I'd see them drip off the bottom of her chin as she put the kettle on or bent to collect the post from the mat at the front door.

Susan seemed to move around without her feet touching the floor. She crept into rooms; she slid out of them again. She cried into her pillow when Phyllis put her to bed. I saw her eyeing the chair at the table where Stephen should be sitting as though expecting he might suddenly appear. I caught her watching me a few times, although what she was looking for I didn't know. I put my hand out to her and she stood beside me, leaning into my side, and it reminded me of standing sentry over Alf when we first got to London. I wondered if she felt the same weight inside, the heaviness of worrying over an adult.

I tried to smile at her, but it felt wrong on my face, felt like I was grimacing.

But Sue smiled back and then she slipped back out into the sunshine to play with an apologetic glance over her shoulder as she left me and I was glad she'd gone.

Phyllis placed the "In Sympathy" cards on the windowsill until she had to start lining them up on the sideboard, there were so many. She read the new ones that arrived each day, salty tears spattering them like rain from her chin, before putting them next to the others.

My own tears wouldn't come.

Not on the morning it happened when the headmistress rang the shop and told us there'd been an accident and that we should come to school, as quickly as we could. Alf flapped his hands at us to say that he'd look after the shop and we drove down the road to the school, not five minutes away, still wearing our aprons. Phyllis clutched my hand in hers as we strode up the path from the school gate, as we spotted the ambulance already there.

No tears came when we got there and the receptionist was crying in the office and someone shut the door when they saw us. But there was a feeling of terror growing in my gut, like a cold hard stone.

Not when the headmistress, Mrs Swanson, took us into her office, white-faced, stricken, and told us that Stephen had fallen from the top of the climbing bars and landed badly.

She said more words, but Phyllis slumped to her knees and it reminded me of Mam all those years ago and that nice young man who asked me to mind his motorbike for him.

In a daze I reached for Phyllis and helped her to her feet when she could stand and the headmistress led us through the school, which smelled of rice pudding and plimsolls, and I could hear the discordant screech of a class somewhere practising their recorders.

Not even when she opened the double gymnasium doors and we saw Stephen sprawled there in the hall, at the bottom of the climbing bars, wearing his gym shorts and white vest. The ambulance people were standing to one side, their faces bleak and their heads bowed, and Phyllis ran past them and fell beside our boy as she cried and cried and cried.

"Would have been immediate," someone murmured.

"A freak accident," said the headmistress, with a small handkerchief pressed to her nose.

"A broken neck," someone else claimed as they gently turned Phyllis away, and she put her hands over her face in horror at what was before us.

And I thought about the other little boys and girls in his class that would have heard him shout, or glimpsed him fall past them. Or even worse, seen him land and not get up again.

Then it hit me, that he'd never get up again. And something turned black inside me, something that felt hard and buried, and I put my arms round my wife to hold her up as I stared sternly before me.

The funeral was on a cold and windy day. Alf shut the shop at lunchtime and pulled the blinds for the rest of the day.

The hearse turned up on time, the driver and another man dressed in black with pale faces, the coffin in the back only taking up half the space. It paused outside the house where Phyllis and I stood on the kerb, waiting to take our place. We walked behind as it crawled up the high street to the church.

Shoppers stopped for a moment on the pavement to watch us walk past, their mouths still and their eyes wide. An old woman crossed herself and a young child stared and sucked a lollipop, and I thought of Susie at home with Peggy the Pie with the promise of custard for tea. It was much better for her to be there than here although, at that moment, I wanted to pick her up, hold her against me and press my face into her tiny shoulder, as it felt like only my little girl could in any way make me feel better. But at only six years old she was with Peggy and had already said her goodbye.

Phyllis and I led the way, Alf on the other side of Phyl in case she needed his support.

But she looked straight in front of her, not paying attention to either of us, her eyes fixed on the small wooden casket. She walked like she had no bend in her legs. Her back was the straightest I'd ever seen it and I knew she was holding herself together, like I'd seen only once before. She had her hand through my arm but it was light as a feather, as though she weren't actually touching me at all.

The market traders walked with us too, the whole market closed for the first time since Christmas Day.

Budgie held a big white cotton hanky forgotten in his hand as he cried openly. I could hear him from the front, gulping and sniffing at the loss of the only chance he had at having a boy.

The others wore their best suits, the ones they had for weddings or funerals, or might have inherited from their dads. They looked like different men to the ones that called out the prices in their overalls and pinnies. The ones that laughed and raised a pint in a salute as you opened the pub door.

The shopkeepers came next. Davey Wenham from the baker, John Rapley from the fish shop. All of the Somervilles from the pub. The Broomes from the garage. The woman from the newsagents and Annie from The Sovs, and I knew it wasn't just because we'd go there after. Even Bert the *Standard*-seller, away from his usual spot at the end of Bridge Street. They'd closed their doors and turned their signs, maybe just for a few hours, but it meant a lot to me.

The schoolchildren and their teachers came last. I was glad about that. I didn't want to see the faces of Stephen's friends and classmates. I didn't want to hear the lighter strike of their school shoes on the stones. I couldn't bear to see the ones I knew – Jason Alexander and Annabel Terry – or the little girl with red hair who lived on the corner. The fact that they were there was enough to undo me. That they were there. And he wasn't.

It was as we turned the corner on the last bit before the church that I first heard the low rumble of a Norton in the distance. Then the closer buzz of a Kawasaki. Next there was the faltering sound of an engine that needed an oil change and I knew that word had spread.

The low noise of another motorbike, then another, and another, filled me with something other than despair. The noise was comforting, like a mother's murmur, or a well-known hymn. I could hear the control in that slow, slow ride, as they discreetly joined the back of the line to pay their respects. The BBC were all there and for the first time I felt my eyes get hot. I knew Stephen would have loved this.

The churn of feeling inside grew as we reached the church gates. We paused for a moment as the pallbearers took the coffin from the back of the car. Perfectly in time, they slid the wooden coffin towards them, and then lifted it on a quiet count of three to their shoulders. It only needed four of them, not the traditional six for a grown-up. Although I knew for a fact that I could carry him myself, just me, as I had done two Saturdays before for a piggyback on the way home from the park.

I heard Phyllis exhale slowly beside me and turned to check her, but her eyes remained glued. To the coffin. The coffin with our boy inside.

We started the walk through the churchyard, the gravel crunching under our feet.

An exhaust spluttered behind me and now I felt it like a punch in the gut. The feeling was moving up inside me, out of my gut and into my chest until it pulsed and filled every inch of my insides. My eyes burned with salty water but my fists were clenched. My knuckles white. Suddenly I realised the feeling was not sorrow.

It was anger. It was a white-hot fury that Stephen was dead. That I'd never ride Josie with my boy. I'd never look to my left or right and there he'd be, giving a quick nod or a lift of a single finger on his grips. We'd never remove our helmets simultaneously and smile after a good ride-out.

I took one look over my shoulder, taking in all those that followed. The old, the young, their faces pinned tightly into place. I scanned right to the back where the BBC were pulling bikes onto stands and removing their helmets and gloves to file in behind us.

And I wished Josie were there, waiting beside them. Because all I wanted to do was turn, run back down the stony path, climb onto her leather saddle, and ride far, far away.

The Everyday

I held tight to the hand that held mine and shuffled behind, through a door. It was darker inside, shaded after the sun and I stumbled into the woman's back, stopped. Was it my room?

"All right love?" she asked over her shoulder before she stepped inside, and I saw it was Phyllis. I wanted to pull her back. I didn't know where we were.

"They do a nice roast apparently," she said and I followed her voice, held on tight, hearing my breath. "I know it's not the Rose and Crown, but this one's closer to your home."

Home? Was I going home?

She sat me at a table and pulled herself in beside me. A big woman sat next to me, trapping me in tight, and a man was on the other side. There were two children. A blond boy and a small girl with no teeth. She grinned at me, all gums, when she saw me looking but then it slid off her face and she played with her placemat. A teenage girl came in last and sat opposite me, eyes flicking about.

I looked around me but I didn't know it. Pictures on the wall. People sitting at other tables. The talking was loud. A man at the next table laughed and rocked on his chair. Why was he doing that? He'd fall. Stephen had fallen at school hadn't he? Someone else slammed their hand on the table and joined in with the laughter. He was wiping his face as though he was crying.

My own eyes got hot. Were they laughing at me? I put my hand to my ear, pressed it there. A knot of something in my gut made me want to close my eyes. Or go home. Hadn't someone said something about home? Phyllis nudged me and I looked at her mouth moving but I couldn't hear what she was saying. She put her other hand on my one, the one holding my ear flat, and lowered it to my lap.

"Bit noisy isn't it, love?" she said. I opened my mouth to say it was too noisy and I didn't like it, but nothing came out.

"Let's get you a drink, shall we, Dad? Fancy a pint?"

Phyllis and the woman were talking. There were wooden ducks on the wall. Billy Sankey's mum used to have them too. They flew up her stairs. Billy and I used to call them Quack and Waddle. Sometimes we used to pretend to be them in the street and run flapping our wings towards the corner.

There was another person, standing at the table, and he was looking at me.

"We haven't chosen yet," the woman said and gave me something to look at. Pictures and paper. I held it in my hands, wondering what it was.

"Oh look, they've got your favourite, Ernie." Phyllis pointed at something on my pictures. "Cod and chips. What do you think of that?" She nodded at me. I nodded back. "I knew you'd love it," she said happily. What would I love? I loved Phyllis. I wanted Phyllis.

The other woman beside me looked like Phyl's mum, Mrs Marshall. But she lived in Margate. They moved there and we got the shop. It must have taken her ages to get here.

The man came back and the woman told him things and they talked. There was another woman at the bar on her own. Sitting up there bold as brass. Shouldn't do that. Not really. Otherwise you'd get called bad names.

The Everyday and Far Away

"Tell Pops what you've been up to," the woman said to the blond boy at the end of the table. He raised his head and stared at me, wide-eyed.

"I got the cup for cricket," he said. His voice high and innocent.

"Isn't that good, Dad?" the woman said at me.

"It's great, really it is, Freddie, we're very proud of you," Phyllis said as if she knew him.

A photo on the wall was black and white. A building. A cart. Nobody I knew. A bridge, a stream. An old car. No motorbikes. I didn't like it in there. We were squished round the table and I couldn't see a window. Walls on all sides. I couldn't see the birds. Or the sky. A corridor out on the far side. My tummy gurgled and felt loose.

"Don't worry Dad, dinner will be here soon," the woman said.

I held on to the cloth. It was Mammy's handkerchief. Then Phyllis took it off me and tucked it into my collar. I pulled it out but she put it back in.

"Just while you're eating," she said and got busy cutting up food on a plate. I looked round for Susie. She hadn't got the hang of a knife and fork yet.

"There you go." And the plate was set in front of me. White, orange and yellow. A big splodge of red. The smell made my mouth water. But my tummy was hurting and I wanted to go home. Back to the house with Phyllis. To sit in our deckchairs in the back garden. We could put the sprinkler on for the children.

The little girl was wiggling around in her seat.

"Honestly, you should have gone before," the woman said and heaved herself out of her seat. They went. They came back, the little girl skipping.

"There's a Christmas concert next week at Dad's home," Phyllis was saying. "Do you think you could make it?"

They talked. I tried to scoop something onto my fork but it moved it around. I tried another piece but it smeared through the red and I didn't want that.

"Let me help," Phyllis said and then I had something in my mouth. Hot. Nice.

"Didn't know it had come to that," someone said and Phyllis shushed them.

I opened my mouth for another piece. Like a baby bird. I chewed. I swallowed.

I lifted my pint, it felt tiny in my hands, and drank a mouthful or two. Phyllis fussed at my chin. The man opposite me raised his pint in a salute.

"Cheers," he said.

I tipped my pint at him and Phyllis wiped the table.

Cheers. They always said that when we went in The Sovereigns off the stall. Even before I could drink, Alf used to get me a half and half after work on a Saturday. We'd have the corner table and Budgie would lay his bets out for the weekend. Annie would shoo us out when it got to teatime, telling us to get home to our wives and mothers. Alf and I didn't have either back then. We'd go home together via the chippy.

The little girl turned up beside me on the wooden bench. She nudged my arm until I moved it and then she climbed on to my lap. I put my arms round her and she sat, comfy as a dog in a bed. She felt familiar. She smelled like lemons. I sniffed at her hair and she laughed at me.

"Stop sniffing me, GrandPops," she said.

The Everyday and Far Away

There was a bowl in front of me then and the girl had to get off. She slid underneath the table and popped up the other side.

"Pop goes the weasel," I said but it didn't come out right. The table was talking again. There were more people coming in the door. Nobody that I knew. Phyllis put something in my mouth. Cold. Creamy. I smacked my lips and people laughed. Patted my chin with Mammy's hanky.

The teenager was looking at something in her hand. Never looked up. The girl whined and got told off. There was a man at the next table with a moustache. Alf had a moustache. My stomach was feeling hot inside and I wanted to be home. My room. The one with the pictures. The one where it was quiet. I put my hands on the edge of the table and pushed myself upwards. I wanted to get up. I wanted to go somewhere.

"Careful there," the man said and stood with me. Something was not right. Something was bothering me. I could hear my own blood in my ears. I put my hands to them.

"You okay, Dad?" the woman said and it was Susie. Her big blue eyes, right there. I wanted to say something but I had a feeling like I was crying and I felt all worked up inside. There was a pressure in me. And I didn't know what to do about it. I looked at the corridor, then at the door. I had to go. I put my hand out towards her, wanting her to take it. To hold it.

"Do you need the toilet, Ernie?" Phyllis whispered and sprang to her feet. She faffed with the chairs, pushing them this way and that so they scraped on the floor. They screeched like crows. She pulled at my elbow and I shuffled out.

"Just this way," she said. "I saw a sign. Excuse me, excuse me," she said to someone's back.

I held her hand. Tried to follow. There was a crowd of people and we were stuck. My trousers flashed hot. Relief surged through me. I breathed out.

"Follow me," she said turning to me over her shoulder. Then, looking at my trousers, "Oh Ernie."

She put her spare hand to her mouth. Flicked her eyes about at the other people around us.

"Could you not wait, love?"

Wait for what?

"I'm sorry, I should have thought. We could have gone earlier. What with you having a pint and all." Her eyes looked so unhappy. Like she'd done something wrong. She was leading me back to a table. My leg was wet and it stung and itched. There was water in my shoe. I plucked at my trousers trying to stop it burning. She picked up Mam's handkerchief from the chair and tucked it into my belt at the front. It hung in front of me like an apron. We had those at the shop. Alf and Son. A family business.

"We'll have to go," Phyllis said to the others, pulling on her coat. "Dad's had an accident."

An accident? What had happened?

"Is Stephen okay?" I said as I couldn't see him, but they didn't hear.

They were collecting bags and the wide woman was off with her purse and the teenager was bright red in the face and looking at the ground.

Nina

Nina stood in the middle of the garage floor and turned in a slow circle, wondering where to start.

She didn't want to throw anything away that might be part of Josie, and that was the problem. She didn't know what was bike and what wasn't out of the various nuts, bolts and stainless steel.

She picked up a cardboard box from the corner and decided to fill it with anything that was definitely not to do with vehicles. That was the easy bit. A bottle of tomato feed, a bug spray, some old newspapers, a seed tray. Soon the box was full. She put it outside the garage door. Next, she dragged out some old carpet and spare floor tiles. She took out a rusty spade, fork with a bent middle prong and a small selection of hand trowels. Some traffic cones, a ramp and a drill. Tins of paint that had Nan's writing on them – *"lounge", "downstairs loo", "kitchen"*. An old clothes horse and a stand for a Christmas tree.

Then she reassessed. It looked like she hadn't even made a dent in the mess. She sighed and drummed her fingers against her thighs.

She moved to the workbench to see if she could safely remove anything from there. A black and white photograph was propped at the back against the wall. It was Pops holding his motorbike helmet under his arm, smiling proudly next to Josie. She held it in her hands for a moment, noticing how young Pops looked, how brown his hair. How big his ears had always been. Then, she studied the bike.

In a flash it came to her. Maybe she could use it to identify the bits? Like the picture on the front of a puzzle box, showing her what the finished thing should look like. Which bits to look out for as you put it together. It was a start at least.

Nina cleared a floor space around her and began.

She glanced at the photo. Black fuel tank. That was easy. Big and straightforward to spot. She lifted it from its resting place and moved it to her new spot.

Another look. Handlebars with black handles? Were handlebars two bars joined in the middle, or one long bar? She googled a picture so that she had a better idea of what she was looking for and then scanned the floor, the shelves, the workbench. Nothing. She looked at the photo again and then realised that maybe she'd jumped ahead of herself. Maybe the grips were separate even to the bar? She looked again – essentially looking for a long, bent, steel bar. Found it, leaning in the corner with cobwebs built from it. When she looked for the grips as individual things, she weirdly found three of them. Maybe he kept spares?

After an hour she had found the larger components of a motorbike. In fact, she'd found more than she needed of certain bits. Two saddles, three exhausts. A fuel tank. Some handlebars and three wheels. The engine was obvious but very heavy so she left it where it was. But it still didn't help with the rest of the garage. The floor remained littered with tiny parts, cogs, metal, tiny chains, bigger chains, pins and rings. She was also aware of the tools amongst the mess that might be needed in reconstructing the bike.

Because that, Nina had decided, was what she was going to do.

When Nan had surveyed the state of the bike, she'd seen it as hopeless. When Nina had opened the door and seen all the pieces – jumbled, scrambled, strewn – the breath had caught in her throat at the prospect of such a huge, complex puzzle to complete. Her fingers had itched to start then and there, her tongue flicked at her lip to get stuck in.

But Nan had been upset by the scene. The fact that Ernie would have been so sad at the state of the bike. Nina had had to delay the onset and take her nan home to Mum's where she had a cry and a cup of tea.

She'd had then to wait a whole day, fizzing and jigging and bouncing before she could get back to it. As she left the house, she was sure she'd heard her mum heave a sigh of relief.

Josie would be put back together. Bit by bit by bit. By Nina. Not only would it make her mum proud of her, but it would make Nan happy. She could even take a photo of it in to Pops.

Nina hummed to herself at the thought. Queen again. "We Are the Champions".

She wasn't stupid, she accepted that she didn't know the first thing about motorbikes, but she'd found a good YouTube channel about motorbike restoration and thought she could follow it on that and maybe work it out. Then she considered if it was maybe all more of a mess than she thought. And if she didn't have all the bits to the puzzle to start with, it was an impossible task.

But she wasn't giving up. She had to do it.

She'd not been able to think of anything else since she'd entered the garage, and it would gnaw away at her until she finished it.

That's the thing with hyper-focus, Nina thought with a sigh, when it kicks in you really can't think of anything else. Like the time with the Rubik's cube. And the time she decided to learn sudoku. Puzzles had always been the thing that got her into that zone. And when she was in it, she couldn't get out of it. Not until the project was complete. Then her attention would stray immediately, and the spell was broken. At that point she was just back to being weird old Nina. But not now.

Frustrated though, she grabbed a pair of secateurs from the shelf and began to cut the stray rose branches that had managed to grow through the top window. Might as well get one job out of the way while she was here. At least it would give her something to tell Nan she'd done. She chopped roughly, letting the plant fall to the floor. The last bit was jammed in the window frame and, as she reached for it to cut it off, a thorn stabbed the soft pad of her thumb and blood immediately beaded there.

Nina stuck her thumb in her mouth automatically, but the blood kept coming. The thought that she was sucking her own rusty-flavoured blood suddenly turned her stomach, so she took it out of her mouth and held it above her head but then the sight of the blood grossed her out, running down her wrist. She yanked open the small wooden drawer in the front of the workbench on the off-chance it might contain tissues. It didn't, but it did have something that caught her eye. A flyer. She picked it up, read it.

First Sunday of the month. Meet at The Sovereigns.

It was the Bromley Bike Club.

The one that Pops used to belong to. In fact, the one he'd started. She wiped her bloody thumb on her jeans and then pressed it hard with her index finger as she read. The blood slowed and stopped as she realised this was what she'd been looking for. The key to her puzzle.

She dialled the number on the flyer for someone called John Palmer. It rang ten times in her ear and then went through to voicemail. She took a deep breath as she waited for his recorded message to end.

"Hello. This is Nina Jackson," she said after the beep, hearing the shake in her own voice as she spoke. Not with nerves, but with excitement. She cleared her throat.

"Ernie Dawes – the founder of your club – is my grandad. And I'm looking for your help."

The Far Away

1974

Turns out I felt angry with Phyllis more than anyone else. It wasn't God I was raging against for taking my son.

It was Phyllis. For not giving me the chance to ride with him. Not once.

Anger was a new feeling in my life, and especially towards Phyl. Other than irritations – her habit of putting cold feet on me in bed, say – and minor annoyances – like her losing her car keys at least twice a week – I wasn't used to being cross with her.

And this was more than that. It was fury.

It didn't fade away as I hoped it would. It grew inside me like it had taken root and was now feeding off my insides.

We tried to make the house more normal – for Susie, and for us.

There was noise again, and school trips and Sunday dinners and picnics in time. We ran the shop and cut the grass and put the bins out. But there was a room with a closed door at the top of the stairs and every time I passed it I felt the knot harden. And grow.

When I looked at Phyllis I wanted to scream. It was unfair of me, I knew, but I couldn't stop how I felt. And once I had to leave the room when I imagined myself shaking her by the two sides of her cardigan. It was so vivid I could see in my mind her head lolling about on her neck.

If only she'd let him ride earlier with me.

If only I'd stood my ground that day and said he was big enough.

"It's your fault I never rode with him," I wanted to shout, to scream. "It was the thing I was looking forward to most in my life."

I caught myself when I thought that. But it was true. It had always been a thought that had shone in the future. More brightly than the thought of his wedding or Susie's engagement when they were grown-ups. With a pull that was stronger than wanting to go to Spain on our first foreign holiday or saving up for a new car.

In my mind's eye we were going to ride the roads together and it was going to be wonderful.

I sat in the armchair next to Phyllis in the evenings, not trusting myself to speak in case I told her how she'd done me wrong. Bad thoughts huddled in my gut, turning and churning until we went to bed and faced in opposite directions for another night.

The funeral director rang to tell us that Stephen's ashes were available for collection. Would we want to have the ashes interred at the graveyard, he asked.

Phyllis was quick to reply. "That's too far away. I want him here with me."

I noticed she said me, and not us.

She bought a vase with a lid, an urn she called it, and filled it with Stephen's remains, and put it pride of place in the centre of the mantelpiece in our living room. He got polished with the other display items, the clock that chimed every hour, the candlesticks from her mother. I heard her talking to him when she thought she was alone.

I entered the room once to find her holding the urn like a baby.

She surprised me then, as her voice shook with as much anger as I had in me.

"You should have let me have another baby," she said, positioning the vase carefully back on the shelf and turning back to me with flint in her eyes. "I wouldn't have cared if he had big ears."

I flinched.

"It wouldn't make up for Stephen though," I said.

"But now we only have one. What if something happens to her?" Phyllis's voice was bitter as she put her hands out wide as though there was danger everywhere in the room. "Then I won't be a mother at all. We should have had another one while we could."

I could only stare as she stalked out of the room and pulled the door shut firmly.

I couldn't reach her. She couldn't reach me.

We were too separate in our grief. In our anger.

Susie stood between us for photographs at family events or days out. It always used to be Phyllis and me at the centre and a child each side. Now, we used Susie as a buffer. On her seventh birthday Susie with solemn blue eyes, with us each holding one of her hands and none of us quite smiling for the camera.

And Josie stayed silent.

Locked safely in the shed, draped in a dust sheet. I passed the chairmanship of the BBC to Davey for the time being and hung Josie's keys on the hook in the kitchen until I could bear to ride her again. It wasn't her fault. I knew that.

It was just the knowing – the knowing that the ride I'd always wanted would never come.

At nine in the evening on Christmas Day, six months after Stephen died, the fire spat out a last flurry of sparks as the last log died and collapsed into the ash.

Susie was already in bed, having ridden her new bike in the garden, and Alf and Peggy were away to the pub, wearing Christmas paper hats and carrying the presents we'd bought them. Old Spice for Alf. A knitted hot-water-bottle cosy for Peg, who suffered with the cold. They'd been wonderful all day, keeping the spirits up and playing Operation with Susie. We'd been glad when they went though, happy just to have survived the first Christmas without him.

Then Phyllis reached across between the armchairs and gently held my hand for the first time since Stephen went.

Her fingers twined through mine, and I glanced at her across the chasm and saw that she was just there, looking at me.

"Why don't you go on the Boxing Day ride-out tomorrow?" she said with a tiny catch in her voice.

I shrugged, not knowing how to say it.

"Stephen used to love watching that. All the tinsel on the bikes." She smiled as though she could see him, running bike to bike, talking to the bikers. "You've not been out on Josie for ages," she added, knowing my last ride was before Stephen died.

"It doesn't seem worth it." My voice cracked slightly as we'd been quiet a while watching the fire, lost in our own thoughts.

"Because he's not there any more?" she said, and when I paused her fingers tugged mine insistently for an answer.

"Because he's never going to be there. Not to ride with me." My voice was sharper than I meant it to be and I heard her swallow.

"I've often thought about that. I made a mistake. It wouldn't have hurt, would it? If he'd ridden on the back with you when he was younger."

My throat closed although something else inside me opened, and I clutched her hand more tightly.

"I'm sorry we didn't have more children," I told her.

She shook her head and I saw a tear fall with the motion.

"I'm not. We had the best two children in the world."

Phyllis leaned over my chair as she passed and kissed me, not quite on my mouth, and my heart tugged inside me, an ache and a swell all at once.

"Coming up?" she said, lifting our glasses from the side tables to rinse them in the kitchen sink.

"Soon," I said, turning my eyes back to the dying fire.

I had an idea.

The Everyday

Lights everywhere. Red ones. Green ones. Silver and gold sparkles.

A tree in the corner of the room. Boxes underneath it. They brought it in and wrapped it up with ribbons and shiny string. Someone clapped when more lights went on.

"Good to see you downstairs, Ernie," someone said. "It's been a while, love."

They sat me down in a chair. I faced the window. The birds were all puffed up outside, feathers fluffed up. The floor outside white and no grass to be seen.

"Brrr," I said.

"Let's get you snug, Ernie," said a man, laying a blanket on my knees. He pushed it all around, tucking me in. It felt nice. He patted my shoulder when it was done.

The birds had a feeder. They hung on it. Clung to it. Sideways and upside down.

"Look who it is," an old woman said next to me. I looked at her and then away. I didn't know her, she had no teeth and I didn't want to see the blackness of her mouth. Other people started coming in. The room was getting full. People were standing round the edges. A man stood in front of the window and I couldn't see the birds any more.

"Mince pie, Ernie?" A woman pushed something against my lips. I shut my mouth, knocked her hand away. What was she doing?

"Maybe later," she said and then moved away.

There were people all wearing red hats. With a white bobble on top. They were lining up near the tree. We used to line up, in the national service. We weren't very good at it at first, but Neddy and I soon got the hang of it. You had to if you wanted to avoid a punishment. I looked at the man nearest me but it wasn't Neddy. Never seen him before.

"They got him out of bed, then," a woman said. "That's good."

"Hello love," someone said in my ear and I started. Face right there. It was Phyllis. She put her hand in mine and I grabbed it tight. Where had she been? I didn't like it when she wasn't there. Her hand was cold and I pulled it under my blanket to warm it up.

"Hi, Dad," someone said and kissed my head. "Decorations look gorgeous!"

"Should we decorate his room, do you think?" I heard Phyllis say, "if he's spending so much time in there?"

"That's a good thought. I've got a little tree that I used to put up in the kitchen. I could bring that in next week?"

Some music started. Drums and trumpets. The old woman with no teeth started swaying about. A man coughed.

"Here we go," Phyllis said. I looked at her. Don't go yet. Please don't go yet. I grasped her hand harder under the blanket.

"Here you go ladies," someone said. Phyl and the woman started eating. It smelled nice.

Phyllis saw me looking and broke a bit off, passed it to me, gently. It was hot, it was pastry. The baker. The butter bits. She wiped my chin afterwards. She looked after me. Like Mammy.

The people were staring at paper, then singing. Phyllis liked to sing on Sunday mornings in the kitchen with the music centre playing in from the lounge. She made the roast and sang all morning, sipping a sherry.

"Don't you look nice, Dad," the woman said when the music stopped for a bit and she smoothed my hair down. Her palm felt nice against my forehead. She was nice, this one. I was tired and wanted to lean my head against her.

"Lost a lot of weight," Phyllis said. But she looked the same to me. Sitting straight in the chair. She looked the same as always. Mrs Marshall.

A robin was on the feeder. I could see it behind the fella's head. It had a bright red fat tummy.

The music started again.

A man behind me cleared his throat. Phyllis shuffled in her seat. The woman the other side smoothed out the paper in her hands.

There was a fanfare and I felt it deep inside me.

"Silent night, holy night," the others sang.

Mam and Alf, sitting by the fire.

"All is calm, all is bright." The voices all together.

Dotty spitting on the logs. Her baby teeth. She wasn't there. The woman beside me had no teeth at all.

"Round yon virgin, mother and child."

I watched Phyllis sing with her whole mouth, just as she had at our wedding. My chest felt tight, like I might cry. She had a lovely voice, did Phyllis. I always liked to hear her.

"Holy infant so tender and mild."

There was a lump in my throat, threatening to choke me. I opened my mouth, to cough, to swallow, but instead a few words spluttered out.

"Sleep in heavenly peace."

My voice was a surprise. I hadn't heard it for so long. It was a bit gruff but it knew what to do.

Phyllis raised her eyebrows as she looked at me and she squeezed my hand tighter between our chairs. I lifted my chin and said again, "Sleep in heavenly peace."

"Well I never," croaked Phyl as she wiped her eyes.

Nina

John Palmer had actually gasped when Nina opened the garage door and stood aside for him to enter. His eyes widened as he took it in and then a grin had spread across his big red face, until he laughed out loud.

"A Norton Dominator," he said, rubbing his hands together in glee. "Well, bugger me."

He shot her a quick glance and grimace by way of apology for his language but Nina laughed it off. She'd heard worse. Her mum was terrible if she burned the dinner.

John stepped into the garage, hitching up his jeans that seemed to want to show his bum crack at all times, not awaiting any invitation, muttering to himself in excitement.

Nina followed, ready to show him the pieces she'd already collected.

But he was already exclaiming as he saw parts, turned them, lifted them, checked their condition, nodding at each new item as though acknowledging an old friend. Then he stood, hands on hips, and surveyed the floor, eyes darting here and there as though searching, finding, moving on.

He'd rung her back the day before, apologising for the delay. He'd been at his son's for Christmas and only just picked up her message. He was happy to have a look, he said, when she explained the problem. He remembered Ernie from years back, when he himself first joined the BBC. He remembered Josie too, he said. Of course he'd have a look.

Now that he'd had that look, he licked his lips.

"What do you think? I'm sure everything will be here, somewhere," Nina said, waving her arms to indicate the entirety of the garage.

John bent over to pick something up from the floor, revealing a shockingly white strip of skin across the top of his buttocks. Nina tried to ignore this as she drummed her thumbs against her thighs.

"Ernie always used to keep her immaculate," he said as he stood again. "He took such good care of her. Used to treat her like one of the family."

"I want to put her together again, so I can show him a photo," Nina said.

"He's a good bloke, your grandad," John said. "How is he?"

Nina felt the fizz building inside her. The last few times she'd seen Pops, he hadn't recognised her. He hadn't spoken. He hadn't really known she was there. It was like he was far, far away now. She missed him already, even though his body was still there.

"Not so good," she said, finally. "Which is why I want to do this now." The fizz was making her want to run around, arms out like an aeroplane. "Before it's too late."

John met her eye, sniffed, nodded.

"Well it would take me a while..." he said, considering. "It's a big job."

Nina thought he sounded like someone quoting for business. A plumber talking about the toilet that needed fixing. Or a builder as they summed up your extension. She stepped side to side, agitated.

"I can't pay you," she said quickly to make things clear.

"I wasn't asking you to," John said. "I just meant it would take time… it's not a simple thing to do. Not for me to restore her properly."

"Oh no," Nina said, horrified. "I don't want YOU to do it."

He scratched his head and it made the zips on his motorcycle jacket clink. "But I thought… You said you wanted my help?"

"Exactly," said Nina. "I want you to teach *me* how to do it. I want to do it myself. Put the puzzle together."

"Hmmm," he said doubtfully, as he looked at the state of the place. "Have you ever done something like this before?"

Nina shook her head, then followed on with a bright, "But there's a first time for everything!" As cheerful and encouraging as she could make it sound. Even to her, it sounded like the punchline of a bad joke.

John moved to the workbench and started grouping random nuts and washers together by size. Was that a good sign? Was he going to go for it? Nina knew she had to let him know what he was in for, before he made a decision. Not just the state of the bike, but the state of her. He had to have the full picture, otherwise it wasn't fair.

"I should probably tell you something before you decide," she said, her stomach hollowing out.

He lifted his eyes to her as he waited for her to speak.

"I've got ADHD." This was a big thing for Nina to say.

He squinted.

She braced herself. It was the first time she'd fronted the information. The first time she'd shown herself as a whole to anybody.

He was still staring as if nonplussed, and she realised he didn't know what she was talking about.

"Attention Deficit Hyperactivity Disorder. It means I have trouble concentrating." She felt her hands fluttering at her sides, as if to demonstrate the point. "It's quite bad."

He flicked a tongue over his bottom lip, thoughtfully.

"But I'm good at puzzles," Nina said, quickly. "VERY good."

He looked around him again.

"And one last thing," Nina went on. She took a deep breath. "I don't want anyone in my family to know what I'm doing. Not until it's done. I want them to think I'm clearing the garage out. I want it to be a surprise."

He chuckled. "What will you do with her when she's done?" he asked.

"Nan wants to keep her for a while. After that I guess she might be for sale if that's what you mean."

If it meant he helped her put the bike together again, Nina was ready to promise him first dibs if that's what it took.

He shook his head.

"No, I've got another idea," he said, tapping the side of his nose. "But let's talk about that when we get there."

She looked at him, hopefully.

"Does that mean you'll help me?"

He stuck a hand out towards her and she hesitated only a second before shaking it.

"I'm in," he said. "Let's get started."

Over the next few weeks, they worked every evening as soon as John got out of work. She'd hear his own motorbike, a yellow Triumph, pull up outside Nan's and she'd be jigging outside the garage door to watch him walk down the path, hitching up his trousers.

The hours went past faster than any Nina had ever known, and she learned a lot. Not just about the bike, the mechanics, the engine, how or why things worked or went together, but things about John himself. The fact that he liked a cup of tea precisely every hour and a quarter and it needed three sugars in it. His wife was from Birmingham and called it a "coop of tay", which John imitated with a laugh. Nina brought a kettle and a supply box to the garage on the second day when she realised just how much he got through.

John swore often and well. It made her laugh. He smelled like oil and aftershave. He had a grown-up son and daughter, and he confessed that he liked them more now that they didn't live at home. He hummed along to the radio, though he never seemed to know the words or the tune. And he never wore a belt for his jeans, even though he definitely needed one.

He also had the patience of a saint.

He pointed things out in a way that she could understand. He showed her useful videos on his phone. He got her to clean the various pieces of Josie and work out how they fitted together. He got her to file away rust. He asked her to oil or grease. He showed her the way the engine came together. The part that each component played in the movement. He showed her how to use the right tool for each and every job. They knelt together on a dust sheet on the garage floor for so long that they creaked when they stood up.

And if he sensed her attention was wandering, he got her to jump up and down on the spot twenty times and sing very loudly the national anthem. Or he'd get her to do press-ups and whistle at the same time. He clapped her on the back when she completed something and grinned like he'd done it himself. They worked long into the evenings, until John's phone would ping with a message from Babs, his wife, asking him if she should give his tea to the dog? Or Mum would WhatsApp Nina and tell her it was time to come home. Then they'd dust themselves off for the night, him seeming as reluctant as her to go.

Nina also learned stuff about herself. She could concentrate better if she took small breaks every once in a while. John's silly challenges also did the trick. At first she'd stalled and felt her neck get hot with embarrassment. Now she laughed as she did them, knowing that afterwards she'd be able to sit down for another hour and concentrate. She found out that no question was a silly question. John always answered them the same. She realised her brain worked well in some ways – she could picture easily in her mind how things moved, how they fitted together, much more readily than she could remember the geographic regions of Africa or the different chambers of the human heart. She didn't mind having dirty hands and short nails even though Jess would have hated it. She liked the fact that her hoodie was handy, for the pockets and to keep her head warm these winter evenings. She concentrated better if she chewed gum because her jaw was busy. She liked learning hands-on, with someone to show her. It was active and fun, and she didn't feel half as jittery as she did in a classroom looking at a whiteboard or staring at a screen. She was enjoying herself, she realised. She was having fun. She was interested.

Every night before they left the garage and locked the door, Nina would cover the parts of the motorbike they'd been working on with a clean dust sheet. She'd whisper goodnight to Josie, or the bones of her, as she turned off the light and then she would realise she was smiling.

The Far Away

1974

Phyllis had raised one eyebrow on Boxing Day morning when I came downstairs wearing my leather jacket and carrying my helmet. She'd been long asleep when I finally got to our bed the night before. She stood, hands in the sink, taking me in.

"Ah, good," she said as I pulled my gloves on.

"See you down there?" I said and she nodded. A proper smile. As though it made her genuinely happy to come to the BBC and see the bikes.

I felt a flutter in my tummy, was this guilt? I left the kitchen, feeling as though she knew what I'd done. It was easier if I didn't catch her eye. It let me think I hadn't done anything wrong.

In the garage, Josie responded as though I hadn't neglected her for months. She kick-started first time; she dropped to a low purr as I pushed her out of the garage. She responded to my every touch, my every lean as I rode her to The Sovereigns.

I realised I was driving cautiously. Lighter with my touch than usual. Gentle on my acceleration. It would take a while to get used to it, I reasoned. I had to give myself time.

I turned on to the high street. Alf heard Josie from his spot outside the pub and turned, hands on hips, as I rounded the corner.

He dipped his head as I pulled up. It looked like a mark of respect and I wondered what he'd say if he knew. What it had taken for me to get here.

It was a good turnout for our Boxing Day gathering. The tradition was that we rode to the coast, where we would park up and drink tea from flasks as we looked out at the horizon and felt the salt wind on our faces. Then each year, we mounted our bikes again and rode back to our houses, our families, and our friends. While we were gone Peggy and Phyllis would spend the day with the children. Boxing Day walks and then bubble and squeak for lunch. It might be harder for them than us this year, with one child missing and just one child swinging between them on the way to the park. But it was definitely going to be easier for me.

The other bikes were already parked down the pavement. The street was full of leather and Santa hats, with pedestrians strolling, talking, comparing. Annie played music out of the pub on to the street. "Mary's Boy Child" and Cliff Richard. She'd have mulled wine waiting for everyone on our return later. But now some of the bikers revved their bikes for the little kids, who put their hands over their ears and pressed their faces to their mothers' legs.

I pulled in to the kerb and dismounted.

Davey waved. Others did too. I lifted my hand, saw the relief on their faces. I was back. I was normal. I might have disappeared for a while because my son had died but now I was back. Doing what I loved best. Riding my bike.

Phyllis and Peggy were at the end of the line. I saw Susie darting between the bikers, calling them all by name, being picked up or tickled by one or another. Her face was unguarded. It was open and happy. She wore a bobble hat with a red pom-pom, and something about seeing her run about as she used to made me want to cry. But I put my hand on Josie's saddle, took a deep breath and watched Susie as she laughed, ran, at last being a child again.

I knew Susie had needed to get back to normal. She needed to be a seven-year-old. She needed us to realise she'd lost him too. He'd been there all of her life. She deserved parents who could look at her without feeling the gap of her brother. She needed to be the best in the family at sport or running or maths without us wondering all the time whether Stephen would have been better. And I needed to be able to hug her close without thinking she'd one day be bigger than him. I needed to laugh at her jokes with a true happiness in my heart. Seeing her now, all freckles and giggles, made me want all of that for her.

Phyllis needed to find a new normal too. I knew she'd never be the same again. Neither would I. Our first-born child was gone. But she must start to feel like she was a good mum. Not just to Stephen but to Susie too. She should be able to relax her back at night and know that she could lean on me. And that I'd be there.

The last few months, I'd not been there. I'd been too angry. The way I'd hurt her made me ashamed.

And I knew I must move forward. To know that, although Stephen was gone, I could find a way of making my dreams come true and of forgiving Phyllis for not letting him ride with me. Because I knew that would be my downfall. It would be the end of us if I couldn't find my way past it.

Last night, watching the fire. I'd accepted everything. It was on me.

The flames licked the last remnants of the logs and took me back to Divine Street. To spitting on the logs with Dot. To Alf, to

Mammy. To Liberty. To the days I'd clean the bike for Alf and he taught me the different parts and how to maintain them.

To the day he pointed to his panniers, and told me he kept his treasures in them, pulling out a boiled sweet, wrapped in sticky paper, for me. Other times it was a satsuma, or a toffee.

Then I remembered Susie as a baby. Recalled that the BBC had put her big, nappied backside into the panniers and she'd stuck there on the side of the bike, sitting upright, waving at us in delight.

"That's one way to take her with us," they'd said.

The fire died slowly. The national anthem played on the TV as the programmes ended and, after the screen went blank, I watched the ash grow cold in the grate. And I knew exactly what I had to do.

Phyllis had been to a Tupperware party in the spring. She'd felt obliged to buy something, she'd said, so had come home with some sandwich boxes and tubs that were now in the top cupboard in the kitchen. The overhead light buzzed as I chose one that I thought was the right size and took it back to the sitting room, turning the kitchen light off again and pulling the lounge door shut behind me.

My hands trembled slightly as I emptied Stephen's ashes from the urn into the plastic tub. For my fingers to be this close to his skin, his heart, his eyes without being able to hug him or muss his hair brought a noise to my throat. A low, low moan. I closed my mouth to keep it in, so as not to be heard, or caught.

The ashes filled the Tupperware almost to the top. Looking at the greyness of it, I thought again how wrong it was, because when I thought of Stephen every colour of nature filled my mind. The blue skies above him as he learned to ride his bike. The red of the berries in the hedge when we went sledging. The green of the new grass in the park when he showed me his handstands, his rolls, his cartwheels.

I tapped the urn gently on the tub to ensure every last flake, hair, cell was in the tub. I shook the tub softly to level it out. Like I'd jiggled his pram a million times to keep him quiet in the shop. I put the lid on and pressed down. It clicked shut on all four sides.

"It's really airtight," Phyllis had said when she showed me her purchases from Jean Evans' party. "Makes it safe for everything."

Only when I was sure it was shut did I take it out to the garage. After I put some tape round the tub to make absolutely sure it would stay closed, carefully I placed it at the bottom of the left-hand pannier behind my saddle.

The side closest to my heart.

I stumbled slightly as I left the garage, thinking of the cold and the dark, but then reminded myself of everything I'd show him, all the places we'd go. All of which would be better than Stephen staying for eternity on the mantelpiece in the lounge.

Back inside, I used the coal scuttle to scoop the ash out of the grate and carefully spoon it back into the vase. I filled it, to the same point, and wiped the outside carefully to remove my dusty fingerprints and evidence of tampering. Placing it back on the shelf, I said a private plea that Phyllis would understand, if she were ever to find out. That she would in fact, one day maybe, approve.

Then I turned the light off and went to bed, where I lay staring at the ceiling until dawn.

Now, Susie tugged at my hand.

"Peggy's going to play Operation with me again, Daddy," she said, swinging on my arm.

"That's good, Susie," I told her, glancing across at Phyllis and Peggy, who were talking to the other wives. They looked ready to be left to their own devices for the afternoon. In fact they were probably looking forward to it. "I'll play you a game when I get back."

Susan bit her lip, cautiously.

"Promise?" she said, and I thought of the times over the last few months that I'd seen her playing in the garden with a ball and had chosen to stay inside. The time I saw her talking to herself in her bedroom, moving dolls about, and I just crept past on the landing.

"Promise." I winked at her and she winked back, perfectly. She'd obviously been practising.

"We off, Ernie?" someone called and I looked at Davey, deferring to him as the new chairman. He nodded and pulled his helmet on as he moved towards his bike. Everyone started their preparations, bikes walked backwards to position, gloves pulled on. I felt the breathless pull of excitement of what I was actually doing as I swung my leg over Josie, and Alf pulled up next to me.

"You okay, son?" he said, holding his visor up so that I could hear.

I reached backwards with my left hand and felt the leather of the pannier there. Pictured its contents, its treasure, and I nodded at Alf.

It wasn't the way I'd ever imagined riding with Stephen. But it was the way it was. And I felt closer to him than I'd felt in six months and I knew I'd go home later to Phyllis, and it would be me tonight that reached for her hand between the chairs.

"Let's go," I said.

The Everyday

"There we go, Ernie," the woman said. "All snug and ready for bed." She stopped fiddling with the front of my pyjamas and helped me to sit back into a chair.

When I was comfy, she pulled a blanket up on to my knees and tucked me in. It felt nice, and snug, holding me there reassuringly. Like Phyllis would have felt in the sidecar when we rode in the winter, her knees under a tartan blanket to keep her warm.

"Let's give your face a wash." She started wiping something damp around my cheeks and, although I ducked and strained, she held my chin and gave me a proper going-over.

"Pah," I said as she stopped. The air made my face cold where the flannel had been.

"That's better," she said, rubbing my face with a different cloth. "Half your dinner round your chops."

Next she picked something up from my chest of drawers and started stroking my head. It was a light scratching feeling that made me want to close my eyes.

"Let's sort this hair out. You look a bit like a mad professor." Scratch scratch scratch. "You know the one in *Back to the Future*?" She nudged me on the shoulder. "That one." Scratch scratch scratch. I felt sleepy, safe, warm. Mammy was good at brushing my hair. She always knew to avoid my ears with the brush.

"There now," the woman said, waking me up. "You just sit there for a moment while I get the bed lowered." She put the black thing back on the chest of drawers and turned the lamp to low. The room was small and in the mornings I could look out to the treetops. I didn't know how long it had been my room. It wasn't in my house, I knew that still. But I came here every night. It was nice enough, I suppose. It had a bed and a chest and a toilet through the door. It had a chair for sitting in and sometimes Phyllis played music in here for me if I didn't want to go downstairs.

"Look at all these gorgeous photographs," the woman said as she headed towards the bed.

The wall she pointed at was covered in pictures. Each one in a frame. Each one different. I peered at them, moving my eyes one face to the next.

A smiley middle-aged woman. A young boy in a black and white photo. He had a missing front tooth and his knees were bigger than his thighs. Looked like he needed a good meal. Then a boy in his sports kit, holding a silver cup. An old man with white whiskers. A bride in a wedding dress. A girl with a Rubik's cube and a big grin. That picture made me smile. She looked naughty, that one. Mammy would have called her a proper little pickle. A picture of me and Neddy Banks in our uniforms, standing side by side with our arms on each other's shoulders. And then a picture in the middle of the collection, of Phyllis. She was sitting at a table and raising a glass of wine at me. The sun was on her hair. I looked at that picture a lot. It made me feel better.

A noise. I turned to the bed hopefully but she wasn't there, in her nightdress, putting creams on her cheeks. Or reading with her bedside light on. In fact there was no bedside light and the bed wasn't big enough for both of us. It was just the woman I'd heard, humming something to herself as she pulled the sheets down.

"Lucky man, you are, Ernie Dawes, look at all those faces smiling at you," the woman said, coming back to my chair. I looked for faces I knew. Where were Mammy and Dot? Where was Billy Sankey and his stinky dog?

The woman held both hands out towards me and, when I put mine in hers, she said, "One, two, three," and I heaved myself up to standing. My legs weren't the same as they'd been once. Now they felt like two little sparrow legs under my bottom and I never quite knew if they'd walk me or not. I let her hold my elbow as I shuffled towards the bed. My ankles felt draughty without the blanket round them.

"And tomorrow we've got porridge for breakfast," she said as she lowered me on to the bed and helped me swing my legs round. She gave me a pill and a sip of water. "Your favourite." Did I like porridge? I didn't know. But she was smiling so I must.

"Not too much now," she said as I drank the pill down, "or you'll be wanting to get up again in an hour or two."

"Sleep well," she said, pulling up the bedclothes. The duvet felt soft as it landed on me. "See you in the morning."

"If you're lucky," I said and it rasped out of my throat.

The woman laughed and put her hand on my head. I wanted her to hold it there for a while.

"Night Ernie," she said.

I moved my gaze to the pictures and it was Phyllis I saw before the light went off.

Nina

Her mum phoned her at about eleven on a Sunday morning. It was her first lie-in for weeks, her first day of rest since starting the Josie Project. She'd spent every waking hour she had free over at the garage since finding the key. The vibration of the ringtone dragged her out of a deep sleep, full of dreams of motorbikes. She fumbled for her phone on the night table as she peeled her eyes open. MUM flashed on the screen. She immediately presumed her mum wanted to tell her of some job she had to do that day. She rolled her eyes as she answered the phone, but when she heard her mum's tired, breathless kind of voice the other end something inside her froze.

"I'm at the home," Sue said on a sigh. "You'd better come in today, love. Sooner rather than later, if you know what I mean."

The silence after the sentence made Nina catch her breath with the weight of it.

She sat up in bed, still staring at the phone, after Mum hung up. She knew what it meant. Pops was dying.

A helpless howl burst out of her as she hadn't shown him the pictures yet. In fact, she hadn't even taken the pictures yet.

They'd only finished the bike last night.

The last pieces of the puzzle put together. The panniers polished and attached to the sides. The saddle buffed and put in place. She'd planned to go to Nan's in the daylight today, wheel Josie out on to the back lawn and take photos that she could show Pops. How beautiful she was. How amazing.

Because she was.

It had taken three weeks of evening and weekends, but Nina had found and cleaned every nut, bolt and screw on that bike under John's supervision. She understood the suspension. She'd tightened the brakes. She changed the sludgy old oil for new, watching it pour like dark treacle. She'd checked the clutch, greased the chain. And then last night, he'd handed her the key.

"Start her up," he said.

The fizz inside of her was almost deafening as she inserted the key. John stuck his thumb in his empty belt loops and nodded.

She'd turned the key in the ignition and they'd laughed out loud as she kicked into life. They took turns revving the engine, marvelling at their work. At Josie.

And now, it was too late. It just couldn't be. She thumped her thighs with her fists as she checked the time.

"Sooner rather than later," Mum had said.

Nina's tummy clenched. Did she even have time to go to Nan's and take the pictures? She'd never forgive herself if she missed the chance to say goodbye to Pops. The reality of it all punched her hard. She was going to say goodbye to her pops. For ever. A million images ran through her head. Him throwing her an apple to catch. Him holding Nan's hand between their armchairs. Him being presented with a certificate at a BBC special dinner that said he was the founder. Him calling her TillyMint. She jumped out of bed.

She might not want to say goodbye to him, but she damn well wasn't going to miss the chance. She couldn't risk it.

She'd ring John and see if he could take some pictures and WhatsApp them to her. The call was as quick as she could make it. John sounded as shocked as she was.

"Leave it with me," he said. "I'll sort it out." And she sighed with relief, knowing that he would. He'd never let her down yet. She pulled her hoodie and tracksuit bottoms on over her pyjamas and was out of the house two minutes later.

Jess and Andy were already there, having dropped the kids at his mum's. They stood by the window of Pops' room, arms round each other. Mum and Nan sat either side of the bed on stiff plastic chairs, each holding one of Pops' hands. Josh was yet to arrive. The room was very quiet and calm, which sent Nina's fizz into overdrive. Was she too late?

She watched as her mum gently wiped Pops' mouth with a wet cloth, and for the first time Nina understood properly the enormity of what was unfurling in front of her.

Pops was Mum's father. Her dad. And he was dying. And one day, she, Nina, would have to go through this with her own mum and dad. She was distraught now at the thought of losing her grandad, but how would she feel at losing her parents? The thought swelled through her chest until it hurt and she crossed the room in a few steps and pulled her mum into a hug.

"Are you okay?" Mum asked into her hair.

Nina nodded fiercely.

"Are *you* okay?" she whispered back and her mum held on tighter but didn't reply.

When Mum let her go, Nina's eyes darted to the bed, then away, then there again and relief rushed through her. Pops was sleeping. She'd made it in time. Just, maybe.

She edged closer to him, moving out of her mum's arms. His chest rose and fell so gently it barely moved the sheets. She could hardly bear to look at him, his face was slack and his mouth slightly open. She could hear the slight wheeze of his breath. She'd seen him sleeping before, sometimes in his armchair at home after a roast at the Rose and Crown. Occasionally in a deckchair on the beach with his face turned up to the sun. This was just the same, she tried to convince herself. This wasn't so scary. She could do this.

She sat on the bed by his legs, conscious of her nan watching her from the other side.

"All right Pops?" Nina said but her voice was weak and weedy. She cleared her throat, tried again. "It's TillyMint," she said, clearer this time. "I'm just here."

She glanced back at Mum, who nodded at her, encouraging her on, but Nina didn't know what else to say. She nudged her phone out of her hoodie pocket and surreptitiously checked it for messages, but there was nothing yet. She mentally urged John to hurry. She might not have long.

"What you doing?" Mum said over her shoulder, but before she had the chance to reply the bedroom door opened again and Josh put a nervous head inside. There were hellos and hugs and then they all changed position so that Josh could take his turn at the bedside. He was wearing his football kit, having been called in at half-time.

"I scored the first goal, Pops," he told the sleeping old man. "Off a header. You'd have loved it."

Nina let herself look at Nan for the first time, scared that she might see her crying.

But Nan kept her eyes intently on Ernie. Her face was sad and tired, but so, so, loving that it made Nina's throat too tight to swallow.

The door cracked open again. Two of the carers, Joey and Mabel, peeked through and raised an eyebrow in Nan's direction. She beckoned them in. Their uniforms were crumpled, their faces were creased.

"We're off shift now for the day, Phyllis," Joey said. "But we wanted to be sure to say our goodbyes."

Nan looked one to the other of them and nodded, reaching out to touch both of their hands. They obviously knew too. They had a lot of experience in this and they thought he'd be gone by morning when they came back in.

Moving silently to the end of the bed, they stood side by side and bowed their heads, almost ceremoniously. A final mark of respect for the man they'd cared for. It was the most moving thing Nina had ever seen. Strangers that knew nothing of the man that he had been. Her pops. The Pops she loved. People who took him at face value – old, incapable – and looked after him as if he were their own grandad, as though he meant something. As though his life counted.

"Thank you," Nan told them. "That means a lot."

Nina forced a swallow and it made a noise. She pulled a fidget spinner from her pocket and whirred and whirred and whirred.

"He's a lovely man," Mabel said.

"A good one," Joey added. They moved to the door, there was nothing else to say.

Joey turned at the last minute.

"Cup of tea?" he asked and as Nan grimaced at the thought of the milky lukewarm tea they served, he laughed. "I'll get someone to bring one up," he said.

Nina's phone pinged. A text had arrived, and she stopped spinning the metal. It was from John.

I thought I could do better than a photo.

Nina frowned and was just about to type back, begging him to just send a picture – and quick – when another message came through.

Come to the window in five minutes. So we know what room you're in.

Nina's foot started tapping and she felt a wave of fizz threaten to overwhelm her.

She breathed in and out slowly, like she'd been practising in the garage with John if her jiggles and flutters were getting in the way of the job she was doing. In for four, out for six. In for four, out for six, just like he'd told her.

"You okay?" Jess said, nudging her, an alarmed look on her face. "You're breathing funny."

Nina ignored her sister and moved close to the window, which looked out to the road and the gravel front car park for the home.

She heard them before she saw them. The rev and roar of motorbikes. Many of them, all together. A ride-out.

When they turned in to London Road, she knew they were coming to the home.

Her breath caught, this time in excitement, and her hands fluttered by her sides like little birds. Like the goldfinches Pops told her he used to have in a cage.

There were maybe thirty, forty of them riding slowly in the middle of the road. Some single file, others two abreast. All shapes and sizes, Triumphs, Kawasaki, BSA, Honda. Harley-Davidson, Yamaha, Matchless and Royal Enfield. Small ones, big hulking machines, hornet yellow, racing green, royal blue. Open visors, full-face helmets, scarves and black leather jackets. And the whole thing led by John on a shiny, black Norton Dominator.

Josie.

"What's going on out there?" Mum asked, standing and joining Nina at the window.

"It's the BBC," Nina said. "They're here for Pops."

Jess and Andy turned to see. Josh left his place at Pops' bedside and stood close enough to Nina for her to be able to smell the sweat of his football match.

The bikes came slowly along London Road, indicators ticking as they approached the home. They filed into the car park, pulling into a semicircle formation, John, front and centre, facing the windows of the building, scanning them all until he spotted them on the top floor.

Nina opened the window her side and nodded at Jess to do the same. The roar and pulse of the bikes filled the air of the room.

Nina turned and found her nan's eyes.

"It's Josie, Nan," she said. "I mended her. For Pops."

Nan stayed sitting where she was, holding Ernie's hand, with a look of amazement as she tilted her face to the windows.

Nina's phone pinged again. John.

Hope you don't mind? The boys wanted to pay their respects.

She waved at him, then typed quickly back. She watched him read the text and then motion to all the other riders, sitting on their bikes, looking up at her family in the window. One by one, they cut their engines, took off their helmets and held them against their chests.

Sue sniffed and Nina heard her gulp back a sob. She put her arm round her mum's shoulders and pulled her in tight. She fitted there well.

The only sound now was Josie. Her engine ran smoothly, without a cough or a splutter. A familiar sound to them all.

The sound of their lives.

Nina glanced quickly at Pops for a sign that he heard it, but he was still asleep.

After a minute or two, John put his hand up in a final wave and nodded at the rest of the group. The engines started again and they moved, like a herd, a group – a family – out of the car park and back towards town.

As the last sound of the motorbikes died, they all turned back towards the bed.

Nan was still at the bedside, holding Pops' hand between her own. Everyone had something to say.

"That was amazing, Neen!" Jess said.

"What a mark of respect," said Josh.

"Did you really mend that bike, Nina?" Mum asked.

But Nina had a question of her own.

"Do you think he heard them, Nan?" she whispered, stepping closer, wanting so much for him to know what she'd managed to do.

Nan hesitated a moment, then patted Ernie's brown-spotted hand and lifted her face.

She broke into a very gentle smile, but it was enough to topple tears down her cheeks.

"He must have done, love," she said. "Because he's gone with them."

The Far Away

1975 onwards

We had almost forty years of riding together, Stephen and I. And it saved me.

We rode the south coast in almost its entirety. We cruised the gentle slopes of Dorset, past a big white chalk man, and along the shingle of Chesil Beach, out to the craggy head of Portland Bill where we heard the crash of the sea on the black rocks beneath.

We rode the cliffs in Kent, the sea far below us, a slate-grey sky overhead. We took in the narrow winding lanes of Cornwall, where spiky trees lined the way. Nothing that we'd ever seen in Bromley. We saw seals in the bays, basking in the sunshine, slinking through the surf.

We went north. To the Lake District where we circled huge masses of water, passing hikers dressed in khakis and carrying maps and water bottles. Past deer that raised their heads at our engines, that watched us as we passed. We stopped in small beamed pubs for a lemonade and a sandwich. We slept overnight in tiny inns where I couldn't stand up straight in the bedroom because the ceilings were so low.

We went with Alf on Libby on a road trip to Wales. Took in woodlands and hilltops of sheep and tiny villages clustered around the mines, where the people sang in church on Sundays and it echoed through the valley, surprising Alf by bringing tears to his eyes. We stopped by quarries and waterfalls and on the sides of pine forests, and smelled the green wood of the cones, the needles on the floor.

We went to the Cotswolds, past stone houses and thatched roofs. We rested by bubbling brooks, by small arched bridges over streams that meandered across green fields. We heard the coo of the doves in painted white dovecotes. We listened to the sound of the river on the stones and the birds in the hedgerows.

We even went to the heart of London. Wanting to show Stephen everything, I rode slowly past Buckingham Palace, purring past the railings, the wall, glancing up at the windows, thinking of our Queen. Past Harrods and Harvey Nichols, and then we rode over Tower Bridge and past HMS *Belfast* on the Queen's Walk. I timed our route past Big Ben to coincide with its chimes on the hour. When the bongs started as we wound our way through rush-hour traffic I smiled behind my visor, thinking how Stephen would have loved it.

We did country and city and village and town. Old ones and new ones and those in between. We did hills and coast and mountain and gorge. We did A roads, and B roads and dual carriageways, avoiding the motorways wherever possible so that I could show Stephen the back ways, the byways and all the things that you miss if you go on the straightest route anywhere.

I spent time with him in the garage with oil changes, greasing the chain, cleaning and changing the filters, checking tyre pressures. I polished the steel, I buffed the leather. We listened to the radio with the garage door open to spring sunshine or closed against winter wind.

We rode with Alf and I treasured that above everything. The three of us out together, side by side. The fact that Alf was oblivious to Stephen being there didn't even matter, because *I* knew.

And after Alf died too, a heart attack one Sunday afternoon watching the football in his armchair, I was even more glad that we'd done it. It helped to soften the blow, the loss of him.

After that we drove out with the BBC on the first Sunday of the month, alongside Davey and Mike and John. The group grew every year and by the time I turned fifty we had as many members. And all of them rode with Stephen just as I'd always hoped.

And as we turned for home every time, as we rode into the close, and I puttered down the drive and into the garage, I'd run my hands over the saddle and pat the panniers and say my goodnights.

Then I'd go back inside and kiss Phyllis and hug Susie, and count my blessings.

Nina

The majority of people had gone. The lines of people wearing black at the church had thinned out before the sandwich buffet at the Rose and Crown, where Nina knew a few faces from the market and the BBC. It was family only by the time they got home and even some of those had gone. Jess and Andy had left to pick the kids up from his mum's as they'd been "too young" for a funeral, and Josh had gone to meet friends at the pub.

It was just Nan and Mum that sank into the sofa now, changed into their pyjamas, black dresses back in the cupboard. They rested their feet on a shared stool, cups of tea on the side table.

Nina had nowhere to escape to, even though the fizz was growing by the minute. She knew she had to give her nan the letter. It was time.

"It was such a good turnout," Nan said, for the tenth time. Whenever Nina had seen her during the day, she'd been talking to someone else, or hugging, or passing a tissue and patting an arm. She'd done the rounds and made sure that everyone who had turned up to pay their respects had been seen and thanked and talked to in person.

"But that was so nice," she kept saying. "All the little stories, the memories that people had. It reminded me of who he was before. Not how he's been these last few years. It helped me remember my Ernie the way he used to be."

Now Nan looked tired but proud. Like she'd done a good job. Nina could only hope she'd was just about to do a good job too.

She felt the crinkle of the envelope in her hoodie pocket, which she'd worn with Mum's consent because it was black. She made herself perch on the footstool even though she wanted to run in the other direction, straight out the back door and onto the trampoline. She took a deep breath, in for four, out for six, and then she opened her eyes to see both women staring at her.

"You all right, love?" said Nan.

She nodded, opened her mouth and then shut it again.

"Been a big day, eh?" Mum said.

Nina nodded again and went for it.

"I found something Nan, when I was clearing out the house," she said, holding out the letter to the older woman.

Nan took it in her hands and peered at the front.

"For Phyllis," she read out loud. "For When I Die in Case I Forget." She frowned. "Top Secret."

She looked at Nina, nonplussed. "What on earth?" she asked and then reached over to the side table for her glasses.

Mum shifted in her seat to be facing Nan, giving her the space to read the letter alone. Nina found her fidget spinner and spun it between her thumb and forefinger, building up momentum.

Nan shook out the page and started to read through her half-moon glasses perched on the end of her nose. She'd only read a couple of lines when she gasped and clamped her hand to her mouth. Nina dropped her spinner.

"What is it, Mum?" Sue said, literally on the edge of the seat.

Nan held her hand up, a stop sign to say they mustn't interrupt, and then she pressed her fingers back to her mouth as she continued to read. Before she reached the bottom of the first page, both eyes had brimmed over with tears that rolled down her cheeks. She brushed them away.

"Oh Ernie," she said aloud and then turned the page. Nina could see the suspense was killing her own mum, who was now trying to read over Phyllis's shoulder.

Nina stood up and jumped up and down a few times, unable to stay still any longer.

Eventually, Nan folded the pages together and looked at Nina very intently.

"When you cleaned the bike out, did you throw anything away?" Nan said in a very low, slow voice as though it was extremely important.

Nina thought about how diligent she and John had been. How they'd used every original piece and discarded nothing authentic.

"No, Nan," she said, emphatically.

"Run out and bring me what's in the panniers," she said with a shaky voice. "A Tupperware box."

Nina knew exactly what she was talking about. She ran as fast as she could down to the garage at theirs where John had left Josie as Nina had asked him to, never happier of a command before in her life.

Her legs went like pistons, her arms pumped the air as she raced down the garden to the garage where Josie now lived. When she returned with the plastic box, Nan was pacing the lounge carpet. Her mouth opened a little but no sound came out as she took it from Nina as gently as a baby and hugged it to her chest. Mum watched her, then flicked a questioning glance at Nina, who was just as bewildered as she was.

Nan sat on the sofa again, box on her lap.

And then, falteringly, she told them what Ernie had done.

How he'd "borrowed his boy" so that he could show him the world and take him on adventures. How he'd apologised for deceiving her with the urn on the mantelpiece, but how their son, he was sure, would have appreciated the ride. Sue made a sound of surprise when she heard what had been put in the urn – ash from the grate.

"Well, I never," she added.

"I know," Nan said. "All these years I've been chatting away to the remains of a Christmas Day fire."

The corners of her mouth twisted and at first Nina thought Nan was going to cry but then a laugh burst out the sides of her lips. Then Sue's eyes began to shine, and both Nan and Mum put their heads back and roared with laughter.

She felt a bubble of something inside and joined in, although not quite sure why, not quite understanding yet.

After a few false starts to get herself under control, Nan finally wiped her eyes again and held out the second piece of paper to show them.

"Look at all the places he took him!" she said, pointing to a few at random. "The Lake District, 1977. Looe in Cornwall, 1986. Petersfield Heath, 1992. Southwold beach, 1996." She blew her breath out all at once. "I've never been to half these places myself!"

Finally, Nan showed them the single photograph enclosed with the letter. It was of Ernie and Alf, with arms round each other's shoulders, standing next to their motorbikes at a beauty spot somewhere in Scotland. Must have been in the early 1990s as Pops still had quite a lot of hair and Alf was alive. Their helmets were resting on their saddles and they both grinned towards the camera, to the unknown photographer, as Ernie reached his hand out to touch his panniers, as gently as Phyllis was holding the contents now.

"I can't believe he did that," Nan said, looking at the list again in wonderment, then raising her face with a smile. "But I'm very glad he did."

"How come you didn't throw it away?" Sue asked Nina, nodding at the Tupperware box. It was scuffed and opaque now with age, and it had some scraggy tape making sure the lid stayed on. It could so easily have been mistaken for rubbish.

Nina thought back to the day she began to polish up the panniers and found the box inside. How John had said he didn't think it was an original piece and the decision of whether to keep the tub had been hers to make.

"Pops always said he kept his treasure in his panniers," Nina said now, "and that's why I couldn't throw the box away even though I had no idea what it was."

"That he did, love." Nan stood up and gave her a kiss on the top of the head. "He always thought you were a very special treasure too, you know. His own TillyMint."

Nina realised nobody would ever call her that again and she needed to go outside to bounce. As high and hard as she could.

When she came back inside, it was just Mum. Nan had gone to bed in her new bedroom upstairs, exhausted.

Sue sat in the corner of the sofa with her feet curled beneath her. A wine glass had replaced her teacup. A Wispa wrapper lay crumpled on the side table. *Line of Duty* was just about to start. She patted the sofa next to her and Nina slid on. Not too close that she'd annoy her mum with her fidgeting but close enough to feel like friends.

"You did so well, Neen," Mum said, pausing the recording to talk. "Not just at the funeral today. But with the whole bike thing. With Josie."

She reached a hand over and rubbed Nina's arm.

Nina wriggled on her seat, already wanting to stand up again. But the warmth in Mum's words, the praise, kept her sitting down.

"John talked to the Norton Museum, Mum," she said. "They'd like to exhibit Josie as an example of a classic motorbike. Make her a permanent fixture in the museum so that people can see her for years to come. They've invited us down to the grand unveiling. If you and Nan agree that's what should happen to Josie."

Mum's eyebrows nearly hit her hairline and she took a decent mouthful of her wine, before shaking her head slowly side to side. "Pops would have been so proud. You really did an amazing job, Nina." She rolled her shoulders back and snuggled back into the sofa, as though taking off a heavy coat.

"And now that Pops has gone, and Nan's moved in I'll have more time," Sue went on, nodding eagerly. "You know, I won't be visiting the home. I won't be popping round to check Nan's okay all the time. I won't be organising funerals." She crossed her fingers on her lap. "And so I'll have more time for you – at the shop and sorting out the college place. You can take that retail apprenticeship by storm." She clenched both fists beside her face and grinned in encouragement.

Nina tapped her fingertips together in a steeple and took a deep breath.

It was now or never.

She had to hope her mum was in a good enough mood with her to take this well.

"Thing is, Mum," Nina said, "I'm not actually going to do that course."

Her fingers tapped a little faster and she stared at them, intently, avoiding eye contact, which would make her want to jump up and bounce about.

"Eh? Well, what you planning on doing then? You can't just work in the shop, you know, Neen. You've got to be in education until you're eighteen. That's the law." Sue pursed her mouth and cocked her head like there was no argument.

Nina shook her head but that wasn't the best move.

"And don't you go looking at me like that, it's not me that makes the rules," her mum added.

Nina was about to shake her head again, but stopped herself, took a deep breath – in for four – then she smiled on her out-breath.

"No, I meant I don't want to do THAT course, Mum. Because I've applied for a different one."

Sue sat up straighter, suddenly looking very like Nan. There was a silence that built inside Nina's chest until her words rushed out to fill it.

"I'm going to be a mechanic, Mum," Nina said, unable to stop her grin, the goofy one that she normally hated. "John owns a garage and he's taking me on as an apprentice, because – as he says – I've got a real knack for it." She laughed, just a little, half-embarrassed, half-proud.

"Mechanic?" her mum said.

"Yep. I'll work four days with John or his guys in the garage, and then have one day a week in college. Working on cars and motorbikes, mending them and putting them back together, just like we did with Josie."

Mum opened her mouth and shut it again.

"It's going to be great," Nina said, as if she knew it already.

"And you've sorted it all out?"

"Signed up at college, and formally accepted the apprenticeship at John's. I start after Easter."

Mum blinked. Once. Twice. Then she gave a small laugh.

"Good on you, love," she said. "Just think. A mechanic in the family." Her smile turned into a hug as she reached across the cushions and grabbed Nina. "I'm really very proud of you," she said in her most "choked-up Mum" voice.

"Thank you cherry much," Nina said into her shoulder as she held on tight.

An hour later, Nina had shown Mum the prospectus page for the course and she'd read about the duration and requirements and pored over the pictures. Then they'd googled John's garage and seen the client testimonials and the five-star rating, and Nina had told her she could get there on the bus and they'd checked the timetable. Then Mum poured herself another glass of wine and remembered *Line of Duty* was still waiting to be watched. Nina stood to go upstairs. She felt the fizz inside, but this time it was a nice feeling of excitement.

"Sleep well, love," said her mum with a tired wave from her corner of the sofa. "See you in the morning."

"If you're lucky," said Nina, softly, holding her eye.

Mum raised her glass to that and Nina went up the stairs to bed.

Ernie

There was a spring in my step that hadn't been there for a while as I crossed the churchyard to the car park where Josie shone in the sun. Her chrome gleamed like my old army boots did after I polished them for hours. Her paintwork shone. The saddle received me like she'd been waiting, cushioning my bottom. I kicked back the stand, took the familiar weight of the bike, held her steady, enjoying the anticipation. Knowing this ride would be the one of my life. Then I turned the key and she sprang into life.

I turned my face to the sun and sat for a moment, listening to the purr of the engine, feeling the vibration beneath me. I revved, lightly, just for the sheer joy of hearing her respond under my hand. To know that she was as ready as I was for one last ride. Her engine pinked, then purred. She was perfect.

The church bells started to ring. A flock of starlings took to the sky from the steeple roof, forming patterns, shapes as they flew over the flowering cherry trees. I watched them, then let my breath out slowly at how beautiful they were. How beautiful it all was.

As their clamouring faded and they moved further away, I heard a new sound, Libby in the distance, the familiar noise of her exhaust. I heard each corner she took and each junction as she came closer and closer until there she was. Alf grinning through his whiskers. His cheeks ruddy with glee. Like he'd just come off the market at the end of the day. The gravel spun under his wheel as he lined up next to me, taking his place. I could smell the salt air on him. It had been so long.

I felt the smile on my own face. It stretched my cheeks wide to see him wink at me. To see the excitement on his face as he prepared to ride beside me.

I felt breathless with the possibilities ahead. The choices to be made. The forks in the road that I hadn't yet taken.

I didn't have a helmet on. I looked at my panniers but there wasn't one attached. I glanced at Alf and realised his own head was bare. His white shock of hair merging with his beard. I didn't need one. Not any more. At last, my ears were free. I'd feel them flap in the breeze as the wind lifted my hair.

The trees dropped dappled shadows to the churchyard ground. The gravestones marked the people that had gone before and I wondered how they'd got there. Whether they all had their preferred mode of transport. I took a deep breath. I was ready. I was exactly where I should be and knew exactly where I was going.

We rode gently, as though in formation, two abreast. There was no rush. No need to hurry. The road was winding and we curved and leaned in synchronised slowness, taking in the new view at each corner, seeing the wonder at every turn. The dewdrops on grass. The berries on hedges. Until we came to the field where the carousel waited. Pinks and reds and blues and greens. A multicolour vision against the green of the countryside. Alf sat back on his saddle and wiped his brow with a handkerchief. My own leg shook as I braced the bike to watch.

Music started and the carousel lurched into life. Creaking metal, flashing lights. I caught my breath as the mechanism gained speed to turn. The candy-pink horse was riderless, as was the aeroplane, and the fire engine with its bell rope swinging in the wind. Nobody sat in the teacup on a saucer, or astride the grey elephant, or drove the police car. But finally, the little red motorbike came round, where a boy in a blue duffel coat held the handlebars, and then lifted his hand in a wave.

This was it.

The carousel stopped and I shut my eyes, waiting for him.

Footsteps crunched behind me on the gravel and I dared not look back. But there was just a slight dip of the wheels as he climbed on behind me and took his position. It was as though he knew how to do it, even though he'd never ridden pillion before.

I knew from his weight, from the last piggyback, that it was my Stephen.

The arms he put round my waist reached right inside me and squeezed my heart. I looked over my shoulder into his eyes, black eyelashes, and freckled nose. I heard the inhale of his breath and saw the bite of his lip and my chest swelled bigger than it had when he was born. The smell of him – the familiar scent of his ever-young skin – the sunshine – made him mine again immediately. It had been worth waiting for. I shut my eyes again momentarily, to hold it tight, to make it last. I opened them again when Alf revved, keen to get on.

"Ready?" I asked Alf, and he nodded.

I pressed the bike forward, and Josie rolled willingly.

"Ready?" I asked Stephen, and he clenched my sides with his hands. His giggle was everything. His smile my guide.

"Hold on tight," I said and we pulled away.

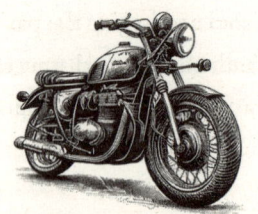

Acknowledgements

Thank you to everyone who bought this secret book to life.

My fabulous cape-wearing agent, Judith Murray and all at Greene and Heaton, for encouraging the 'passion project'.

All at Oneworld and most especially my editor, Jenny Parrott, who fell hard for Ernie and championed him all the way, crying as she did so.

My copy editor, Jacqui Lewis, who was brilliant as always.

I couldn't have written about Liverpool without my long-time friend and Northern expert Anne Jackson, the original TillyMint.

Similarly, I couldn't have written about Norton Dominators if my dad hadn't lived and breathed vintage motorbikes, until dementia took him off to the faraway before his death in 2019. See Dad, I was listening.

To Euan, for always and everything.

Thanks everyone. I couldn't love this book more.

Reading Group Questions

1. How did you find the author's writing style? Was it easy or hard to read and how long did it take you to get into the book?
2. Although Ernie plays the central part in the story, there are a host of other characters involved. Who was your favourite character and why?
3. Which character did you empathise with the most and why?
4. How realistic did you find the relationship between Ernie and Nina? How does it compare to your own family relationships with grandparents or grandchildren?
5. How did the book relate to your own life? Did it evoke memories or create connections for you?
6. Did you find it engaging that Ernie's significant life stages were told through his love of motorbikes? If you were telling your own life story, what would be the theme or vehicle that would carry it though?
7. What was the most memorable scene in the book for you and why?
8. How did you feel about the ending?
9. If you could ask the author one question about their book or their reasons for writing it, what would it be?